Praise for the Book From Prominent Orthodontists and Other Dental Specialists

"Timely and insightful, this profound work is brilliant in its simplicity. Dr. Lauson cuts to the core, outlining the real connection between the human airway, mouth breathing, crooked teeth, TMJ disorders, and latent disease. Straight Talk about Crooked Teeth clearly outlines how to achieve the coveted movie star smile with a deeper understanding of how debilitating conditions like obstructive sleep apnea, ADD/ADHD, bedwetting, and headaches can be avoided. It is refreshing to finally have these important lessons and concepts in one easy-to-understand book for every parent, patient, dentist, and physician who really cares about straight teeth, healthy TMJs, quality of life, and longevity. Colleagues, it is time for my beloved dental profession to not only change lives with a winning smile, but more importantly, to SAVE LIVES!"

J. Brian Allman, DDS, Noted author and lecturer
Diplomate, American Board of Dental Sleep Medicine,
American Academy of Pain Management
Director, TMJ Therapy and Sleep Center of Nevada,
Elite Dental Institute—www.EliteDental Institute.com
Online Sleep Academy—www.OnlineSleepAcademy.com,
Reno, NV

"The book Straight Talk about Crooked Teeth should be mandatory reading for every orthodontic provider in the United States and Canada. This book should also be read by every parent contemplating making an orthodontic investment in his or her child's future health and well-being. Its principles embody the fundamentals of what is necessary for long-lasting, highly cosmetic, and highly functioning results, which if not followed, will result in only a compromised solution to the presenting orthodontic problems. I can only pray that Dr. Lauson's treatment principles will seep deeply into the conscience of the world's orthodontic profession."

Brendan C. Stack, DDS, MS, Orthodontist, noted author, and lecturer
Vienna, VA

"I have personally had a very similar understanding and conclusion regarding the current state of orthodontics. The concepts so clearly presented can help patients avoid unnecessary extractions of permanent teeth and jaw surgery. I commend Dr. Lauson for his efforts to advance orthodontics in a more functional and stable manner than traditional orthodontics allows. To think more and do things differently than the conventional wisdom, teachings, and methods say marks true progress. We can provide superior results for our patients by evaluating each of them as a whole system, a complete person, not just their teeth. It is my hope that this book and Dr. Lauson's thinking become the mainstream in orthodontics; then orthodontics will have a great impact to improve the attitude, self-esteem, and overall health of people everywhere. I highly recommend Straight Talk about Crooked Teeth!"

Lloyd Truax, DDS, MSD, Orthodontist, author, and lecturer
Founder and 1st Chairman, Mayo Clinic Orthodontic Department
Rochester, MN

"Dr. Kent Lauson's book, Straight Talk about Crooked Teeth, is an excellent resource for parents, patients, doctors, and dentists. Dr. Lauson clearly explains the connection between a beautiful smile and the keys to overall health. Dr. Lauson is a university-trained specialist in orthodontics and has spent his career building on this education and finding synergy from related medical and dental fields in order to more effectively help his patients. Now these years of study, work, and real-world application are set forth in an easy-to-understand guide. When followed, the principles that Dr. Lauson describes will not only result in maximum facial aesthetics, but also the best foundation for lifelong optimal health. I have spent my career helping people who suffer with TMJ problems, facial pain, and sleep apnea. I applaud Dr. Lauson for publishing information that I know will help many people avoid such problems and help parents make informed decisions that will help their children avoid such problems later in life."

Jamison R. Spencer, DMD, MS, Noted lecturer and author
of Small Airway, Big Problem: How Sleep Apnea
Often Goes Undiagnosed in Women, Children, and Skinny Dudes
President, American Academy of Craniofacial Pain, Diplomate, American
Board of Craniofacial Pain and American Board of Dental Sleep Medicine
Boise, ID

"Dr. Lauson has done an excellent job of integrating the orthodontic-TMD-sleep connection in the treatment of his patients. This book clearly illustrates why orthodontic clinicians must embrace the functional, nonextraction philosophy. Failure to deal effectively with TMD and sleep apnea with our orthodontic patients can result in serious health problems in the future. I would encourage all clinicians who want to diagnose and treat holistically to read this book. Dr. Lauson shows many successfully treated patients throughout the book. It is a must read for patients as well as all orthodontic clinicians who want to improve the quality of their patients' lives."

Brock Rondeau, DDS, Noted author and lecturer of orthodontics,
TMJ dysfunctions, and dental sleep medicine
President, Rondeau Seminars
Ontario, Canada

"It is nice to finally see an orthodontic text written in patient-friendly language that comprehensively looks at the entire craniofacial complex and not just the fit of the teeth. For dental professionals and patients alike who are interested in the intimate relationship between teeth, jaw joints, muscles, airway, and posture, this book is a must read. Clearly and concisely put together, Dr. Lauson has made a strong case for the use of functional facial orthopedic techniques and the 'nine keys' to not simply create a prettier smile, but to have long-lasting, positive effects on the overall health of the individual in ways not often associated with dental treatment. Straight Talk about Crooked Teeth *will be prominently displayed in our reception and consultation areas as an invaluable piece of patient education."*

Dan Demmings, DDS
British Columbia, Canada

"I would recommend this book for any parent contemplating orthodontic treatment for his or her child or any adult who is unsure which brace option is the best for him or her. This book dispels some of the myths associated with 'traditional orthodontics,' such as 'don't treat till the child has all his or her adult teeth' or 'extractions of premolar teeth, to resolve crowding, is the ideal treatment solution.' This book is long overdue as it also links the medical/dental interface, e.g., nasal airway obstruction, TMD, snoring/OSA, and

maligned jaws. Dr. Lauson must be applauded for his continual search for answers beyond the confines of his traditional training. His results speak for themselves."

Derek Mahony, BDS, MDSc, Orthodontist and international lecturer
Sydney, Australia

"*Spot on! This is the book every mother should read before choosing an orthodontist for her family. Most practitioners doing orthodontics don't pay enough attention to the airway and TMJ. The nine keys to lower facial harmony should be part of every graduate orthodontic curriculum. Why not have a more beautiful smile while opening the airway, alleviating headaches and clicking jaws, and improving posture. A must read for every parent, dentist, and orthodontist.*"

Michael Gelb, DDS, MS
Clinical Professor, NYU College of Dentistry
New York City, NY

"*Dr. Lauson has completed a timely and wonderful book for the orthodontic patient, as well as for the orthodontic practitioner. His many years of experience have enabled him to develop a system for optimal orthodontic treatment. A full smile that retains all permanent teeth and creates an optimum airway is the enviable goal for orthodontic professionals and their patients.* Straight Talk about Crooked Teeth *is a must-read book.*"

Ron Cook, DDS, MSD, Orthodontist
Educator, Next Generation Orthodontic Education
Lake Havasu, AZ

"*This easy-to-read book, specifically aimed at the layperson interested in learning more about options for orthodontic treatment, is written with simple explanations of orthodontic and scientific terms that keep the reader engaged. It presents relevant, reliable information that will help patients and parents choose the best orthodontic options through informed decision making. Dr. Lauson challenges some outdated concepts, using orthodontic literature to support his assertions. The information is presented in a balanced, well-thought-out manner, which most fair-minded people will find easy to accept. I highly recommend Dr. Lauson's book* Straight Talk about Crooked Teeth *to anyone who is contemplating orthodontic treatment."*

G. David Singh, DDSc, PhD, BDS, Lecturer and author
of *Epigenetic Orthodontics in Adults*
Director, Smile Foundation
Beaverton, OR

"In all my years in dentistry, I have never seen a book like this; certainly nothing out there is comparable at this time. This book is a "possibility" book— showing that beautiful life changes are possible as a result of the treatment that Dr. Lauson has to share. He has shown that even the most complicated of cases are treatable with predictability when the principles in the book are implemented. I would recommend this book to anyone."

Jay W. Barnett, DDS, FACD, Orthodontist, noted author, and lecturer
Former Chairman, L.D. Pankey Institute Orthodontic Program
Parker, CO

"Dr. Kent Lauson's book Straight Talk about Crooked Teeth *hits the nail on the head. As a functionally trained TMJ dentist who has instructed thousands of dentists worldwide, I wholeheartedly agree with the powerful concepts put forth in this book. The Lauson System is clearly explained, and if it's treatment objectives are followed, it will not only allow the creation of beautiful smiles, but will enable treated individuals to live much more healthy and happy lives."*

William B. Williams, DMD, MAGD, MICCMO, Lecturer and consultant
Founder, Solstice Dental Advisors
Atlanta, GA

"I give this book two big thumbs up! A well-written and concise guide for people considering orthodontic treatment for their children or themselves; this book not only teaches, it also engages you to read more and understand that there are better ways to accomplish results holistically than traditional methods allow. Dr. Lauson has taken a complex set of ideas and techniques to

develop a system that is easy to follow and has excellent results. The multiple aspects of total health as they relate to orthodontics are truly inspiring and are vital information for everyone. The cases presented show the evidence-based results as well as the quality, compassion, and commitment he gives his patients and the years he has spent refining his craft. In my thirty years of working in the orthodontic industry, I have seen many changes and learned a great deal. This book has given me new energy and proves that the envelope is ever expanding; I'm enthusiastic to share this with others. Dr. Lauson is an advocate with an important mission; keep it up."

Kevin Truax
President, Tru-Tain Orthodontics
Rochester, MN

"Dr. Lauson has produced a timely book that was written for parents and patients, which helps them to understand the relationship between the head, neck, and in particular the mouth as it relates to the general health of the individual. He is a professional who has incorporated this holistic approach into his orthodontic practice as it relates to health in general."

David T. Grove, DMD, MS, MSEd, MSc, Orthodontist
Associate Professor of Orthodontics, Next Generation
Orthodontic Education
Las Vegas, NV

Testimonials from Patients Who Have Been Treated by Dr. Lauson

"I want to share my experience of what Dr. Lauson and his 'expander' technology have done for my little girl, Riley. We were referred to him by our dentist when Riley was six years old because of an overbite. I told Dr. Lauson that she was asthmatic and that we were desperate to get her weaned from her daily medications. He noticed dark rings under her eyes and inquired if she had allergies. He commented on how small her mouth was and asked if her tonsils and adenoids had been removed. I told him that she had them removed because of a sleep apnea condition, which helped but did not eliminate the condition. He commented that in addition to correcting the overbite, the expander would change her life. It would not only correct her overbite but would also dramatically open her nasal passageway, making it much easier for her to breathe through her nose. This then could have a profoundly positive effect on her asthma and sleep apnea conditions. Now, over a year and half later, Riley no longer takes any asthma medicine. She has a beautiful smile, and she no longer has sleepless nights from sleep apnea. She plays soccer and can play the length of the game without needing her inhaler at all. I am so blessed for the changes she has experienced by this technology. I want to thank Dr. Lauson and his staff at Aurora Orthodontics & TMJ for Riley's life-changing treatment."

—Kris W., Parent of Riley (Child Patient), Bellevue, Washington

"When I was younger, I was embarrassed by my teeth and never wanted to show them when I smiled. I had a very small mouth with too many teeth that were all messed up and turned around. Dr. Lauson's treatment has completely changed my life. Today my teeth look beautiful. I am more confident in myself now; I love to laugh and smile and show off my teeth. I can never thank him enough for everything he has done for me."

—Brittany E., Teen Patient, Aurora, Colorado

"Dr. Lauson not only gave my daughter a beautiful smile, but more importantly, he gave her self-confidence. She didn't smile much because she didn't like the way her teeth looked and when she did smile, she kept her lips closed. I will never forget the day she got her braces off; her smile was amazing. I could see her smile in her eyes for the first time. She had so much more than just pretty teeth: she stood taller and she was so much more confident in everything she did. I cannot thank Dr. Lauson enough for what he gave my daughter."

—Mother of Brittany E., Aurora, Colorado

"My underbite caused me to feel extremely self-conscious. I had pain that went from behind my ears, all the way down my neck and shoulders, and down into my back. My sister found Dr. Lauson and called me one day. She said, 'Cathy, you have to see this doctor. He's absolutely amazing! He does everything naturally—no surgery, no drugs. He will fix your bite, get you out of pain, and give you a nice smile again.' . . . I was completely impressed with the whole process: with his philosophy, with the staff. I had talked to previous dentists and they told me that the only way to fix my jaw and my bite was to break my jaw and have it wired together for six to eight weeks; I knew there had to be a way to do it naturally without having to go through a surgical procedure. The holistic approach that Dr. L. takes is pretty incredible; I had been told before by previous doctors that once you're an adult you can't expand your palate. So I thought, 'Are you sure you can do this?!' When I got my expander, and it started moving, it was amazing. Dr. Lauson's staff is incredible. It's like a family environment around here. They just make you feel so at home. Everybody in the office, from the front desk to all the girls in the back, really cares about what's happens to you and how you're progressing. Dr. Lauson is phenomenal. You can just tell he's a very compassionate, caring man who really wants you to get the best treatment. I tell all my friends and family that he's the first person I've ever been to that really wants to take a holistic approach to fixing my bite and fixing my jaw. I'd recommend him to anybody."

—Cathy H., Adult Patient, Aurora, Colorado

"I highly recommend anyone who is contemplating having orthodontics done to see Dr. Lauson. I now travel from the east coast for my visits since I moved from Colorado during my treatment. The office is phenomenal, and I'm so happy to be here and to be one of Dr. Lauson's patients. It really has been a great experience."

—Rita B., Adult Patient, Gaithersburg, Maryland

"The office is beautiful, and it's always a fun place to go."

—Teen Patient, Aurora, Colorado

"I was so excited to learn that an orthodontist utilizing neuromuscular concepts was available to me and my daughter. I knew that the appliance my daughter had in her mouth (placed by another orthodontist) was not allowing her joints to have full range of motion. Now both of us are being treated by Dr. Lauson! We are both thankful to have found him!"

—Dr. Lori K., Patient and Parent of Teen Patient, Boulder, Colorado

"When I came in I had pretty severe headaches, and I couldn't open my jaw at all. I had ear problems, sinus problems, and postnasal drip. I think Dr. Lauson is working on the whole problem—not just straightening my teeth—so that as I get older, I won't continue to have gum problems and headaches. I've seen what he's done and have a huge trust factor with Dr. Lauson."

—Mary J., Adult Patient, Aurora, Colorado

"Now, after treatment, I no longer have symptoms. I got really lucky that in my second time in braces I ended up here. It would be nice if every orthodontic office knew how to do these procedures because there'd be so many more happy people out there. If there was a way I could tell everybody that needed braces or jaw repair to come here, I would! I really didn't want to believe that everything Dr. Lauson was saying would come true. It sounded too good to be true; but the truth is, it was true, and it just took time to see that. He really knows what he's doing!"

—Seth K., Adult Patient, Centennial, Colorado

"I had a huge underbite. Other dentists said they would have to break my jaw, but I didn't have to have surgery to fix my jaw; Aurora Orthodontics had another solution."

—Isaiah, Teen Patient, Aurora, Colorado

"The treatment here has been a miracle for me; with my symptoms, it's really been life changing. I feel better, and I'm able to live a healthy life. I love this office and I think anyone would love coming here. It's very clean and professional. The staff is wonderful and they really do care."

—Jennifer S., Adult Patient, Littleton, Colorado

"Well, based on my family's history of having nice teeth, I figured I would be the same; that turned out not to be the case. As I grew up, I began to feel out of place at family events, even when just hanging out with my friends. Finally my mother had enough and decided that my teeth needed fixing. I eventually saw that she was right. I noticed that in all my photos that I never once smiled. But after having braces, for once in my life, I actually feel happy and am able to smile about it!"

—Ricardo B., Teen Patient, Denver, Colorado

"Braces were not something I was looking forward to, but after seeing the final result, I am so happy I went through the process. I would like to let other kids know that having orthodontic treatment is definitely worth the wait, and you'll be very pleased with the outcome."

—Ashlyn S., Teen Patient, Aurora, Colorado

"We feel fortunate that Dr. Lauson and his caring team were recommended to us for our child's orthodontic treatment. A smile can leave a lasting impression and is often the first thing others notice and remember. It was important for us to be able to provide our child with the proper orthodontic care in order to give her a smile that she could be proud of. Dr. Lauson's dedication to improving our child's smile has made a vast impact on how she interacts with others. It has given her confidence and pride in her appearance. We appreciate his area of expertise in expanding the palate to create a beautiful, full smile."

—Parents of Ashlyn S., Aurora, Colorado

"*The transition in my mouth has been pretty incredible, and I'm excited about the finished product. I'm amazed at the wonderment of enjoying a meal, enjoying the flavors and chewing my food to the level that it actually digests better. A whole new world is opened up to me. I've worked with lots of service organizations throughout my life, and generally when I work with a group over a period of time I always find the flaws. I have yet to find the flaws in this organization. The people here are the most caring, loving people.*"

—Dennis P., Adult Patient, Redwood City, California

"*When we first met with Dr. Lauson, we explained to him that my son had special physical concerns. He recommended expansion of his upper jaw rather than removing teeth or surgery. The treatment that he performed had the added advantage of not upsetting the relationship of the jaw and teeth to the spine, and it addressed some of the sinus pressure he had been experiencing as well. Because my son had cranialsacral work done, his body responded especially well to the expansion and better than any other option we looked at. Dr. Lauson's time frame for treatment was fantastic. It was such a quick process because the palate adjustment made the time in actual braces minimal. The team Dr. Lauson has put together is excellent and helps to make the trips to Denver from Jackson, Wyoming well worth it. The before and after changes in my sons photos are dramatic. The fact that this was accomplished without surgery and tooth extraction, previously recommended by other professionals, is a tribute to Dr. Lauson's judgment and experience. I personally appreciate my sons beautiful smile. We are forever grateful for Dr. Lauson's fine work.*"

—Sherry F., Mother of Nick (Teen Patient), Jackson, Wyoming

"*I had a narrow jaw and my teeth were not matching. The enamel was chipping off my teeth because of the way they were matching up . . . All the symptoms I had when I came in are gone. I don't have any of the headaches, my jaw doesn't hurt anymore, and the tension in my neck is gone. My smile is a lot better than it was, even though I didn't start for cosmetic reasons.*"

—Jennifer O., Adult Patient, Aurora, Colorado

"*The understanding that I have of Dr. Lauson's process of treatment is that it is based on scientific, traceable evidence and conservative treatment philosophy. No big mystery, just a gifted understanding of the processes of the human body and how it works. If you are searching for an answer, which you are if you are reading this . . . trust me . . . HERE IT IS!! I will always be an advocate of Dr. Lauson's treatment because it has changed not just my mouth, but also my quality of life. Who knew how much pain had taken away from me? Thank you, Dr. Lauson, you have made a huge difference in my life.*"

—Susan S., Adult Patient, Littleton, Colorado

STRAIGHT TALK
about
CROOKED TEETH

STRAIGHT TALK
about
CROOKED TEETH

THE NEW ORTHODONTICS

**Learn about The Lauson System and what
you must know to get that "Movie Star Smile"
without extractions or surgery**

S. KENT LAUSON, DDS, MS,
ORTHODONTIST

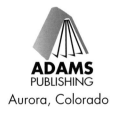

ADAMS
PUBLISHING
Aurora, Colorado

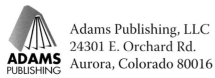

Adams Publishing, LLC
24301 E. Orchard Rd.
Aurora, Colorado 80016

First Edition

Printed in the United States of America on acid-free paper.

Publisher's Cataloguing-in-Publication available upon request

Hardcover: 978-0-9839620-0-7
Trade Paperback: 978-0-9839620-1-4
Ebook: 978-0-9839620-2-1

Photo credits: Judy Galusha, Judy Birschbach, and office staff
(All photos on the cover and cases shown are taken of patients treated by Dr. Kent Lauson)

Book Consultant: Ellen Reid

Cover and Book Design: Patricia Bacall

Editor: Jillian Harvey

Disclaimer

For over twenty-five years, I have proven to myself the validity of the treatment methods and new goals for orthodontics brought forth for the first time in this book. The material is presented in a way that the average nonmedical professional can understand. Much of the material that is presented herein is nontraditional and, therefore, may not be accepted by the establishment of university training in orthodontics. The traditional establishment training of oral maxillofacial surgery may also not accept these teachings, as many of the techniques used negate the use of surgery and show results, in many cases, that are as good as or better than what has traditionally been accomplished with surgery. As this book is widely read, it may impact how orthodontics is performed in the future. Some of the nine keys to lower facial harmony presented will be more readily accepted than others. Three of the keys are already widely accepted, but the other six are not. Many progressive orthodontists have already accepted most, if not all, of the keys. However, no one, to my knowledge, has presented all nine keys in a concise, well-defined pattern as is done in this book.

Although the nine keys represent my current thinking, I am not implying that these are the only keys that may exist. There may be other keys that I don't currently recognize or that others may come up with now or in the future. All works of science are invariably incomplete works. It is important to understand that I am not a university professor or a research scientist. This information is derived from my own clinical experience as an orthodontic specialist and from what others have shared through lectures and writings, which may not be the same as what other orthodontists have experienced. My intention is to write additional books, as time allows, which will probe more deeply into the subjects of adult orthodontics, permanent solutions for TMJ dysfunctions, and permanent solutions for obstructive sleep apnea. These books will also expand the concept of the nine keys to lower facial harmony.

Legal Disclaimer: This book and its contents do not prevent, diagnose, or cure any disease or condition. This text is for educational and informational purposes only. If you or any person has any of the conditions talked about in this book and are looking for help to solve a disorder, please consult a medical or dental professional with expertise in your area of concern. The professional that you consult with may or may not have adequate knowledge and experience to follow the treatment ideas spelled out in this book. The opinions expressed in this book, although well thought out over many years, are only my opinion. I have attempted to be accurate and thorough in my explanations at every level, and I (along with anyone involved with the publication, distribution, or sale of this book) assume no responsibility.

Table of Contents

PART III: THE LAUSON SYSTEM: CASE STUDIES

Foreword

I appreciate very much the honor and trust Dr. Lauson has afforded me by allowing me to review his book, *Straight Talk about Crooked Teeth*. This is a phenomenal book! It is so easy to read and can be enjoyed by adult parents of patients as well as dental and medical professionals. This book is a "possibility" book—showing that beautiful life changes are possible as a result of the treatment that Dr. Lauson has to share. I would recommend this book to anyone; the complex systems and concepts presented here are explained and demonstrated with a clarity that allows the general public to easily understand, while also piquing the interest of the dental and medical professional who would be inclined to venture here. In fact, I believe that this book is so instructive that it should be used as part of the curriculum of graduate orthodontic programs everywhere.

I am especially impressed with the case studies chosen that exhibit the use of The Lauson System. They are all actual patients treated by Dr. Lauson and show the wide variety of the treatment concerns that can be addressed by understanding the Nine Keys to Lower Facial Harmony that he writes about throughout the book. He has shown that even the most complicated of cases can be treated with predictability when these principles are implemented.

In all my years in dentistry, I have never seen a book like this; certainly nothing out there is comparable at this time. Another book, *Epigenetic Orthodontics* by Jim Krumholz, DDS, MS, and David Singh, DDS, PHD, was recently published for dental professionals. Dr. Lauson references this book in *Straight Talk about Crooked Teeth*, as it supports many of the concepts of his book. The fact that both of these books are available tells me that the dental/orthodontic community is ready for a paradigm shift in thinking that will result in much better patient care. Enjoy the book and become informed and enlightened. You will be much better equipped to receive optimal patient care.

Jay W. Barnett, DDS, FACD
Orthodontist, Parker, Colorado
Noted author and international lecturer
Former Chairman, L.D. Pankey Institute orthodontic program
Faculty member, multiple university dental schools

Acknowledgements

This is a book that I have had in my head for a good number of years, but to actually get it completed is a task that, any author can tell you, is more involved than one can imagine when first starting. It, like any other calling a person accepts, was just something I had to do. However, I am sure it could not (or would not) have been completed without the support of many helpful people. I guess that is true of any meaningful accomplishment. I am deeply indebted to the really fine people I acknowledge here:

I am grateful for the immense help of my very talented assistant, Sharon Gilmore. She has been a pillar in the effort to produce the book, always seeing the vision and never being afraid to corral me in when I have gone astray. She helped with all the early editing, was the person I went to most often to bounce ideas off of, and was indispensable in communicating with other parties concerning many aspects of the book. A great many thanks to Ellen Reed, my book shepherd (really!), who guided me through the complex maze of book publishing and was a great inspiration to produce the finest book possible. Patricia Bacall, a creative marvel, is to be thanked for all the design and layout work, outside and inside, giving the book a beautiful look. My fine editor, Jillian Harvey, is so detailed with her work; I swear she could find that needle in the haystack. Thanks for seeing things that go past the rest of us mere mortals. Others who helped with editing along the way include (especially) Sharon Carr, who influenced my emphasis within the book, and Pamela Guierriera, who did early editing work with the book. Many thanks also to staff members

Christian Wrenn, Holly Baller, and Trish Westin, who gave me valuable feedback after reading the original manuscript. I also want to thank my fine professional photographers, Judy Galusha and Judy Birshbach, whose portraits grace the book cover as well. Many thanks to Kathy Boucher and Todd Gilmore for the great illustrations. Matt Curtis, my social-media guru, deserves much praise for website and SEO development. I am lucky to have the backing of my publisher, Greenleaf Book Group and Emerald Book Group, and the professional people who I am working with there, including Tanya Hall, Justin Branch, Jessica Foster, and Julie Prien.

I want to thank many of the fine doctors who have had an influence on my way of thinking, some of whom also have written endorsements for this book: Drs. Wick Alexander, Brian Allman, Larry Andrews, Jay Barnett, Ginny Baker, Leonard Coldwell, Norman Cetlin, William Clark, Michael Dierkas, Paul Dragul, Rolf Frankle, Harold Gelb, James Gerry, Tom Graber, Barry Glassman, Dwain Grummons, Bill Harrall, Egor Harvold, Robert Jankleson, Marcel Korn, Jack Konegni, James Krumholtz, Earl Ladder, Roger Levin, Alan Lipkin, James McNamera, Larry Price, Mariano Racabado, David Singh, Jamison Spencer, Terrance Spahl, Brendan Stack, and Lloyd Truax.

Many others have also shown their support in one way or another. Special thanks to my sister, Clarice Cryder, and her husband, Mike, and all their children and grandchildren (twenty-one at last count). Thanks to the rest of my very understanding staff: Liz Miscles, my great personal assistant; Brianne Noelle, marketing and PR; Tamara Burhenn, my talented lab technician; Jenny Taylor, clinical coordinator (over twenty great years now); Billie Simmons, Jessica Smith, and Eden Herrera, great clinical technicians; and Sue Campbell and Donna Garrett, who beautifully handle front-desk duties. Thanks to many personal friends who showed great encouragement: Douglas Allen, Nick Wadhwani, Jim Fleming, John Czingula, Lee Rindner, Bob Brehm, Chuck Mastin, Vicki Machanic, Barbara Frackowiak, Lynn Schriener, Ann McGirty, Cynthia Forrest, Lori Kemmet, Jennifer Miller, and Bonnie Holden.

PART I

EVOLUTION OF FUNCTIONAL FACIAL ORTHOPEDICS

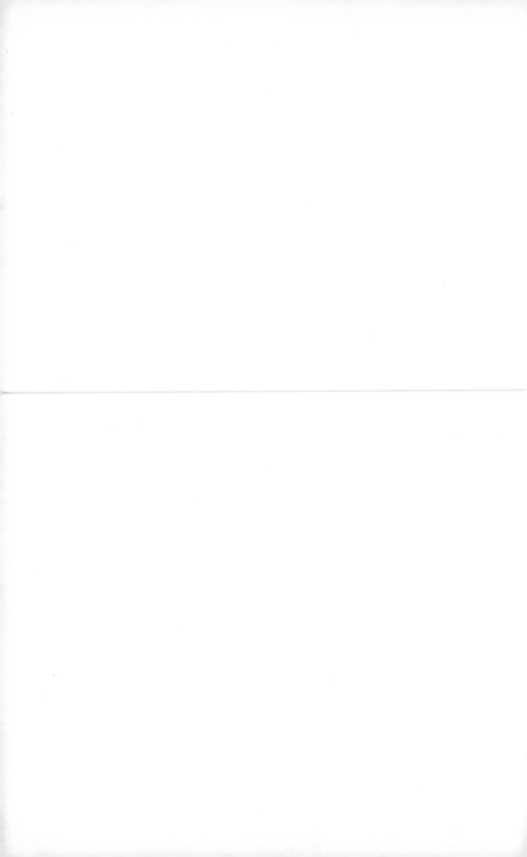

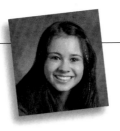

CHAPTER 1

Great Smiles Are a Huge Asset in Life!

A growing child is really a wondrous thing to behold. All children have the potential to be whoever they want to be in their futures. One may dream of being a highly esteemed professional, a teacher, a lawyer, an accountant, or a doctor. Another may dream of being a famous actor, a musician, or of having a great family. As long as children keep their dreams alive, they have the likelihood of achieving them and more.

A good parent always wants the very best for his or her child and certainly always has the child's best interest in mind when making daily decisions. How children develop into teens, and then into adults, is affected by what they personally believe about themselves; in other words, their self-image is critical to their success in every stage of life. A beautiful, healthy smile is a gift parents can give their child that will have a positive effect that can last a lifetime.

How important is a great smile? It is no secret that having an engaging smile is a huge advantage in our society. Several studies done by the American Academy of Cosmetic Dentistry reveal the impact orthodontics can have in a person's life:

- 99.7% of Americans believe a smile is an important social asset.
- 94% of those polled said when meeting someone for the first time, they are more likely to notice a person's smile over attributes such as eyes, height, or figure.

- 96% of adults believe an attractive smile makes a person more appealing to members of the opposite sex.
- 74% feel an unattractive smile can hurt chances for career success.
- Only 50% of all people polled were satisfied with their smiles.

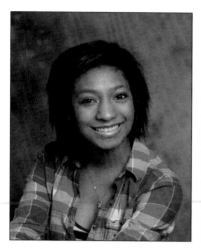 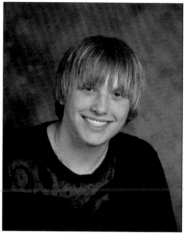

These photos of actual patients of mine exemplify the type of treatment results routinely seen with use of The Lauson System.

When asked, "What is the first thing you notice in a person's smile?" the most common response was "the straightness of the teeth." Because misalignment of teeth is the most common physical defect within the human face, how lucky we are to have a ready answer to this problem: The neighborhood orthodontist has the solution we are looking for.

This book, *Straight Talk about Crooked Teeth,* is not only about the fine practice of orthodontics, but also about how this specialized field of dentistry is destined to evolve far beyond its current emphasis of simply creating straight teeth and a pretty smile. As you will soon see, the teeth have an influence far beyond the mouth, and movement of teeth has farther-reaching implications that can affect a person's overall health and well-being. The information presented here will inform the reader of these implications, offering not only warnings, but also presenting solutions to greatly improve the quality of one's life in ways that go far beyond having a great smile.

THE EVOLUTION OF A TREATMENT PHILOSOPHY

The catalyst for a change in this approach to dentistry began in a rather unexpected way. There I was, the newly appointed preventive dentistry officer at a small US Air Force Base outside of Kansas City, Missouri, telling a young airman (like a private in the Army) how to take better care of his teeth. They really were a mess and my job was to teach him how to floss and brush his teeth properly to prevent dental and periodontal disease.

I showed him plaque (taken from his mouth) by putting it under a powerful microscope and showed him all the dangerous bugs growing between his teeth and under his gums. I thought, "Boy, if this doesn't convince this chap to take better care of his mouth, nothing will." I felt some frustration, as it became apparent that I wasn't getting my valuable points across, when he unceremoniously blurted out, "Doc, I really hate my teeth! I just wish they would go away!" Wow, I was really taken aback by his self-effacing comments, and I could see that if he kept up the direction he was headed, he would most certainly get his wish. His brash, but truthful, statement had really blown the wind out of my sails. However, he really got me thinking. If I couldn't motivate someone who didn't like his teeth enough to take care of them, then all the instruction in proper prevention of dental disease was just a waste of breath. The answer was in helping people feel better about themselves by giving them smiles they could feel great about.

During the next couple of years, I came to the realization that teeth can be beautiful or they can be ugly, depending on a person's perception and a number of other factors. I also began to understand how dentistry is both an art and a science and can affect a person's entire self-perception. This cemented my resolve that I really wanted to be involved with enhancing the appearance of people's teeth. I wanted to help transform smiles from being unattractive to being something that people would be proud to share. At that time, the movement in cosmetic restorative dentistry was just in its infancy, so I equated a beautiful smile with "straight teeth." I decided to become an orthodontist so I could straighten people's teeth and help them be proud of their smiles.

A BRIEF HISTORY OF ORTHODONTICS AS A SPECIALTY

A little bit about the history of orthodontics is in order. Even though dentists had tried their hands at straightening teeth several decades before, orthodontics first became recognized as an actual specialty of dentistry at the turn of the twentieth century. In 1901, Dr. Edward H. Angle started the very first specialty program for orthodontics at the Marion Simms College of Medicine in St. Louis (which later became St. Louis University Medical Center), the specialty program I had the privilege of attending. Even in the early 1900s, controversy was brewing. Dr. Angle was a strong advocate against the removal of permanent teeth when performing orthodontics; however, others disagreed and it became a hotly debated topic. But in the 1920s, Dr. Charles Tweed, a persuasive teacher at the time, gave arguments in support of extractions, which have been very influential in the academic world over many years. This philosophy, however, has lost more and more appeal in the last few decades as nonextraction techniques have come more into vogue.

TRADITIONAL ORTHODONTICS DEFINED

Throughout this book I use the term "traditional orthodontics," which is what the majority of orthodontists do when they perform their work. This differs from the kind of treatment advocated in this book. My definition of traditional orthodontics is as follows: orthodontic treatment methods as taught by most university graduate programs throughout the United States. These traditional methods include an emphasis on the use of braces or fixed appliances (see Appendix A for description of all treatment appliances) to straighten teeth with very little use of removable treatment appliances, which have been used predominately in Europe. However, there are exceptions and some schools do go beyond the traditional approach to include a more functional approach, but because most schools are typically traditional, a high percentage of the brain power in academia has gone to using and improving the braces and not into other less traditional approaches to straightening teeth.

There is nothing inherently wrong with improving an important aspect of orthodontics, such as braces, except that it can be shortsighted to place almost all of the emphasis on teaching braces, while excluding the more holistic removable treatment appliances that have been used in Europe with great success. As you will see, braces are only part of the treatment equation and are limited in what they can do.

In thinking through why this has occurred, I have come to the conclusion that orthodontics, like many other areas of medicine, is influenced by a number of large corporations who sell their products to the private practice orthodontist. Simply put, these corporations make braces, wires, and other devices to move teeth. They are motivated to make better braces and convince the orthodontists to use them in order to beat out the competition and increase their profits. The treatment philosophy I am advocating does nothing for these companies, as removable treatment appliances are typically made in small, local orthodontic labs. These removable appliances cause positive changes in the bone structure and work in conjunction with the braces to move teeth.

Most trained in traditional orthodontics have little experience with this concept, and consequently, few of them use these appliances effectively. In recent years, the notable exception to the discussion about braces has been the advent of clear aligners, namely Invisalign® (see Appendix A for description of all treatment appliances). This remarkable invention is having a major influence on orthodontics today. Although Invisalign is a true megatrend in orthodontics, it is important to know that not all orthodontists use Invisalign and that aligners cannot accomplish some of the facial orthopedic changes talked about and shown in this book. They can, however, produce some orthopedic changes and can replace braces in the majority of instances. It is interesting, however, that Invisalign, which Align Technology produces, is also backed by a corporation with stockholders. This fact, along with effective advertising, explains why the general public is so aware of the brand name Invisalign. We will discuss this important advance in more detail later in Chapter 12.

MY PERSONAL EVOLUTION

My own university orthodontic training was traditional in nature. I followed accepted traditional treatment protocols that routinely called for the extraction of up to four permanent teeth when dental crowding was present. This treatment also included surgery to correct skeletal imbalances when indicated. During this time, I participated in dental study groups that included some family dentists, and quite often the question arose regarding why orthodontists were removing so many permanent teeth while treating patients. My answer was, "Because without extracting these teeth, the stability will not be good." My orthodontic education had taught me that Dr. Charles Tweed experienced instability with his nonextraction approach and achieved better results with the extraction of up to four bicuspid teeth.

In spite of my somewhat-programmed response, I began feeling more uncomfortable with this answer and started to question my own treatment philosophy. I began to understand how changing the bone structure can impact not only the process of moving teeth, but also the stability of the final result, making full, beautiful smiles possible without surgery or removal of any permanent teeth. In looking back at Dr. Tweed's initial nonextraction approach, it turned out that his treatment wasn't stable because he didn't expand the jaw's bone structure before he placed braces on the teeth, thus causing later instability of the teeth due to the lack of bone support. I, therefore, advocate the enhancement of inadequate bone structure prior to braces.

As I stated before, braces alone are only part of the treatment equation and are limited in what they can do. I have realized over the years that the result of traditional orthodontic thinking has, in many cases, left the patient with a compromised long-term result.

"Whenever you find yourself on the side of the majority,
it is time to pause and reflect."
—Mark Twain

TMJ DYSFUNCTION IS A FACTOR

The recognition that TMJ dysfunctions (TMDs) could be caused or prevented depending on how orthodontic treatment was performed was another growing concern. The temporomandibular joint, or TMJ, is the complex joint in front of the ear that allows the lower jaw to move in order to chew and speak. Orthodontists routinely have to deal with the troubling question of what to do about those patients who experience the sometimes-painful symptoms of TMD either before or during orthodontic treatment.

I was uncomfortable with the limited training and lack of knowledge received about this condition at my orthodontic residency program. The university orthodontic specialty programs did not, and still do not, give much training in this very important area. This may be due to the fact that there is continued controversy about what the proper treatment of TMD is. In other words, many dentists still don't agree on the proper treatment even though treatment for TMD can be highly predictable and effective if properly completed. My best advice to the reader is the old adage "buyers beware." Do research on who has a reputation for consistently getting great results.

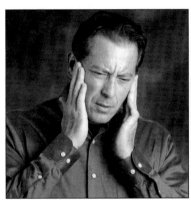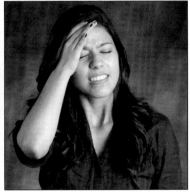

Controversy has existed for many years concerning the idea that orthodontic treatment can actually cause TMJ dysfunction. Although I believe improper orthodontic treatment can cause TMD, proper treatment can help in its correction if already present and can prevent future TMD if certain principles talked about in this book are followed. It is up to the individual orthodontist or dentist to gain the knowledge of how to effectively prevent and treat TMD.

This is an area that orthodontists and dentists must become competent in. I personally believe that if a problem exists before or develops during treatment, the doctor doing the treatment should have a solution for the problem. However, symptoms of TMD may not appear until years after orthodontic treatment. At the time of treatment, the condition can be subclinical (not readily apparent), but is, nonetheless, developing. As orthodontists, we should be in the business of preventing disease as well as curing it. This is an area that can see great improvement in the coming years as many of the answers to treating these challenging conditions are currently known by many dentists who have taken the time to study TMD treatment.

IN SEARCH OF ANSWERS

I continued to search for answers beyond the confines of my traditional training, and this was when my journey began to turn and pick up speed. In pursuit of knowledge, I averaged eighteen trips a year over the next five years to complete over two thousand hours of much-needed continuing education. Much of this education was outside the fields of orthodontics and dentistry in other related fields such as otolaryngology and even chiropractics. I looked at little-known side effects of malocclusion (improperly fitting teeth), such as poor head posture, to gain a better understanding of the possible effects of my treatment that reached beyond the mouth. I welcomed the most challenging cases because they motivated me to find better solutions to problems by continually asking myself, "Is there a better way to do this treatment?" and "How can I achieve better results?" During the most recent twenty-six years of practice, I have applied the knowledge I've gained from the successful treatment of thousands of patients, which provides a basis of support for the holistic philosophies and powerful treatment techniques referred to in this book.

"To raise new questions, consider new possibilities,
to regard old problems from a new angle, requires creative imagination
and marks real advance in science."
—Albert Einstein

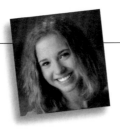

CHAPTER 2

Limitations of Traditional Orthodontics, Two Case Studies

In today's society, people have the opportunity to do research on the Internet in virtually any field, including medicine and dentistry. This is very good news; no longer do they have to take the word of their family doctor or dentist or rely on them for all the answers. They can take a much more personal responsibility for their own health, which has far-reaching implications. The informed patient or parent can have a more active role in deciding a course of treatment.

In my orthodontic residency, I was taught that some orthodontic problems are too extreme to be treated with braces alone. Our primary option was a helping hand from the friendly oral surgeon. Cutting and repositioning bone structures allowed us orthodontists to move the teeth into a more desirable position with braces. There was not much mention about the side effects of surgery (of which there are many). The following is an example of how an informed consumer was able to make a better choice for his child.

AN ORTHODONTIC CASE: SURGERY OR NOT?

Sally, a fourteen-year-old girl, and her physician-father traveled from northern Wyoming to my office for a consultation. Her upper jaw was substantially narrow and the treatment offered to her previously was not to her father's liking. The only option presented by several local orthodontists was surgery to widen Sally's upper jaw, and after healing for six weeks, she could then be treated with braces. Her doting father knew there had to be a better way and was happy to find that there was. Even though they lived in another state, her father felt the six-hour drive to my office was well worth the sacrifice for the health and well-being of his daughter. As a physician, her father was amazed when I recommended functional facial orthopedics using a simple orthopedic expansion appliance (see Appendix A for description of all treatment appliances) used for a six-month period—and was perplexed that other orthodontists had not recommended the same procedure.

After the treatment was performed and had gone so smoothly, he commented half-jokingly that he wondered if there was some sort of a kickback in place between oral surgeons and orthodontists for recommending surgery rather than the procedure I had used. I assured him that certainly wasn't the case and also informed him that virtually all orthodontists, myself included, had been trained that way. Specifically, we were taught that the bone structures of the upper jaw were fused together after about age twelve. Widening this bone structure traditionally required a surgical procedure that involved cutting through the bones above the teeth to spread out the upper jaw. This is one of several traditional treatments still being taught that can cause unnecessary damage to the patient. The following testimonial letter from the actual patient's father is presented in its original form:

> Our visit to the local orthodontist was not a positive experience. My daughter was told that her "condition" was quite serious and that it was vital that this be corrected soon and that braces initially would not come close to addressing the problem. The orthodontist stated that anyone who said that this could be done any other way was a charlatan. His treatment consisted of reconstructive surgery, upper and lower jaw, at his estimated cost of $40-50,000. After this he would apply braces for an additional charge of $8,000.
>
> My daughter was extremely distraught. I became acquainted with Dr. Lauson through a mutual acquaintance; however I was told that his practice was in Denver, a distance of 700 miles round trip. An

appointment was made and the situation was explained. My daughter was overjoyed and pleased that the surgery would not be needed.

Fast-forward one year: I can't believe the changes that have been made. Her smile and her dental alignment look 100% better. Her confidence has blossomed, and it seems as though you made an impression as she is considering the dental profession, and more specifically to become an orthodontist. Thanks again for your help: consider this another success story.

Dr. Daniel A.,
Gillette, WY

This story is not an isolated incident by any means, and it points out that limited thinking still dominates the traditional training for orthodontists. It is time that the university specialty programs and practicing orthodontists accept the use of certain holistic treatment regimens that can drastically reduce the need for surgery.

ANOTHER PROBLEM CASE: TMJ DYSFUNCTION

Michelle, age forty, came to my office after suffering for many years with severe headaches. She also experienced severe jaw joint pain; eye and ear pain; ringing in her ears; hearing loss; substantial clicking; grating and locking of her jaw joints when she ate food; and a myriad of other painful and debilitating symptoms, all of which helped to confirm a diagnosis of TMD. Over several years, she had unsuccessfully sought help from a number of doctors and therapists.

Her dental history revealed that she was missing all four first bicuspid teeth. At age fourteen, she was treated with a traditional orthodontic approach in which those four teeth were extracted to address crowding that was present at the time. She also had a severe overbite. At the time she consulted me, years later, some crowding had reappeared since the constriction, or narrowness, of her jaws had not previously been addressed and instability of her bite remained.

Twenty-six years after her initial orthodontic treatment, Michelle wondered if there might be a connection between her clicking jaws and the painful headaches that had plagued her for so long. After taking necessary x-rays of the jaw joints and completing a thorough evaluation, my answer was a definite yes. X-rays revealed that her jaw joints were significantly out of alignment. Her lower jaw was posteriorly displaced—that is, not in a normal, healthy position. This was likely the jaw position she had prior to her first orthodontic treatment, but her orthodontic treatment did not correct the problem at the time. This, more than likely, was due to the fact that a thorough evaluation of the temporomandibular joints was not done at the initial exam and an awareness of the developing problem was not apparent.

Over time, the posterior displacement of her jaw caused an impinge-ment of the nerves and blood vessels in the back part of the jaw joint, so it became painful every time Michelle bit down to chew food or to swallow. These nerves and blood vessels go to various areas of the head, including the eyes, ears, and even the brain. Also, over time, a piece of cartilage called a disc, which helps to create smooth movements of the jaw joint, migrated forward and got pushed out of the normal position by the improperly functioning lower jaw. As Michelle chewed, the disc going in and out of a normal position caused the clicking sound. We needed to correct these problems.

Treatment of her jaw joints lasted about six months and included the repositioning of her jaw to an ideal position using a neuromuscularly balanced mandibular orthotic (see Appendix A for description of all treat-ment appliances) on her lower teeth. We determined the correct position and treated the muscles with gentle electrical pulses. Neuromuscular massage therapy treated the larger muscles of her neck and was also performed in our office. During this time of approximately four months, her symptom levels were reduced by over 90% (meeting our treatment objectives), so we could move forward with the second phase of treatment. Over the next six months, we used expansion appliances to broaden both her upper and lower dental arches, followed by the final phase of twelve months of braces to correct her teeth to match the healthier jaw position. This gave Michelle the happy result of a beautiful smile with a normally functioning jaw. Her symptoms were virtually eliminated and remained so five years after the completion of her treatment. Michelle wrote the following to share with you her thoughts regarding her treatment:

When I was fourteen, I began the orthodontic process with another orthodontist. My teeth were extremely crooked due to crowding and I had a severe overbite. This orthodontic process included the removal of four teeth to make 'room' for the over-crowding. I wore the braces for approximately eighteen months and was moved into a retainer. I wore a removable retainer for approximately four years and a cemented retainer on the bottom teeth for approximately ten years. I enjoyed straight, beautiful teeth for many years until I began experiencing pain in my left ear. I visited my regular doctor who referred me to an Ear-Nose-Throat specialist who ran a series of tests and could offer no relief. At a routine visit to my dentist, he mentioned that my ear pain could be a result of TMJ and that I should visit an orthodontist. I did some research and found that Dr. Lauson was well known for providing adult TMJ treatment, so I made the appointment and after consultation with Dr. Lauson, began treatment in 2006. Since going through the treatment, I have gone from the high range of the discomfort scale to almost no symptoms.

Michelle

The two cases presented illustrate the importance of a proper, comprehensive evaluation (including TMJ function) and orthodontic/orthopedic treatment. Shortsighted treatment is often recommended. Second opinions can be valuable, especially when treatment involves irreversible procedures such as orthodontics or surgery. Making sure the doctor has the experience and knowledge to use noninvasive functional facial orthopedics, and not just braces, can make all the difference in the outcome of treatment. If too much emphasis is placed on treating patients with just braces, the removal of permanent teeth or surgery is more likely. Additionally, ignoring the effect on the TMJs can have long-term, negative consequences.

> *"Some men look at things the way they are and ask why?*
> *I dream of things that are not and ask why not?"*
> —George Bernard Shaw
> (famously quoted by Robert F. Kennedy)

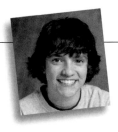

CHAPTER 3

Functional Facial Orthopedics: An Idea Whose Time Has Come

This is the part of the journey where the answers to my questions and the knowledge I gained began to take shape. In previous sections I have described some of the limitations with the way traditional orthodontics is performed in the United States. This section will provide the solutions as I see them. My solutions are expanding (pun intended) the way orthodontics is performed, giving both the patient and the dental practitioner performing orthodontics a better idea of what can be expected from these progressive orthodontic techniques. Although not widely used today, many of these goals and techniques are not new and did not originate with me. Their importance, however, has compelled me to put them together in a concise form called Nine Keys to Lower Facial Harmony.

The phrase Functional Facial Orthopedics (FFO) has been coined to describe a critical part of the treatment used to accomplish these nine keys to lower facial harmony. If we defined FFO as anything that influences the facial structures to either grow or to change structurally, it would have to include influences such as environmental effects (like airborne allergens), adverse habits, or even a person's genetics. This would be much too broad of a definition. A more restrictive and more accurate definition is as follows: Functional Facial Orthopedics (FFO) is the effect of applying therapeutic gentle pressures to reshape facial structures or to reposition them to improve the health and appearance of an individual.

THE SURGERY DILEMMA

Without FFO, virtually none of the lofty treatment goals described herein would be possible, and this book wouldn't have been written. Furthermore, the creation of nine keys to lower facial harmony would be pointless because their goals would be out of reach. You might ask, "But couldn't these goals be accomplished with a combination of braces and surgery?" The correct answer would be absolutely not! Orthodontists and other dental practitioners often look upon surgery, with its attendant costs, patient skepticism, limitations, and side effects, as a necessary (but last) resort. No orthodontist would suggest doing surgery on almost every patient. Fortunately, with proper knowledge, FFO can and should be performed on almost all patients safely and successfully. People usually come to the orthodontist because of crooked teeth. The reason for crooked teeth (or dental crowding) is generally because of constricted jaw structures; therefore, a dental bone structural imbalance is present, necessitating FFO. Because of the many drawbacks of surgery, especially when weighed alongside the hesitancy of many patients and parents, many times surgical treatment plans are not followed through with.

This constant battle in the mind of the traditional orthodontist— whether to recommend surgery or not—is a battle I am sure he or she would rather not fight. This dilemma is one of the reasons why there are so many problems created with the traditional orthodontic approach. It is also a very big reason why the orthodontist should work at solving these skeletal problems with noninvasive FFO. A huge opportunity exists in changing our way of thinking.

"Think Different."
—Steven Jobs

Unfortunately, many orthodontists don't realize that they have the choice of a very potent treatment option in FFO. They haven't been taught enough about the techniques to be comfortable with them, so they don't really understand what they are missing. My hope is that this book will change all of that. Once they know that it *can* be done, they may be open to learning *how* it can be done.

I have put a number of challenging cases in this book to emphasize how very well they can be handled with FFO techniques to create broad and healthy smiles, thereby avoiding surgery and extraction of permanent teeth. I have also included a couple less extreme cases to show the value of using FFO in treating more-straightforward problems, which are also much more common, to turn an okay smile into a dazzling one.

HOW DOES FFO WORK?

Essentially, bones change over time due to pressures being placed on them. You may be familiar with the ancient Chinese custom of binding young women's feet so that they didn't grow past a certain point. Well, the same principle of pressure-induced or restricted growth applies in facial development. That is why adverse oral habits, such as thumb sucking, can create facial skeletal growth problems. It is also the primary principle in orthodontics itself, allowing an orthodontist to do his or her job: straightening teeth. Teeth move within bone structures because of the pressures exerted on them. FFO uses these same principles, but the pressures are very broad, exerting influence over a much larger area than a single tooth.

Remember our definition of FFO: *the effect of applying therapeutic gentle pressures to reshape facial structures or to reposition them to improve the health and appearance of an individual.* This does two things:

First, it corrects bone structures that are narrow or underdeveloped by expanding or enlarging them to bring them into harmony with the rest of the face. Virtually all of the bone structure problems seen are due to underdevelopment. This is where FFO shines and expansion can generally be accomplished within about a four- to six-month period.

The second type of correction is to reposition bone structures, usually by moving the lower jaw forward. While the upper jaw is being expanded, the lower jaw can come forward on its own as it is no longer trapped behind the upper teeth. The use of an FFO appliance, called a bite plate or bite ramp, can also be used to guide the lower jaw forward. This creates a better balance with the rest of the face. A more advanced method of repositioning the lower jaw involves a very specialized type of appliance called a mandibular orthotic, which can correct a TMD by moving the jaw into a more ideal functional position.

Generally speaking, FFO appliances are most commonly used on the maxilla (upper jaw). As show below, with the use of slow palatal expansion (SPE), truly remarkable changes can be made in the upper arch.

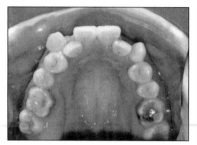 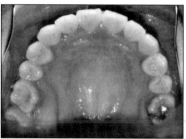

This shows the roof of the mouth of a teenager treated with FFO (using SPE) to expand the upper jaw, then braces.

By contrast, an appliance called a rapid palatal expander (RPE), which is still commonly used in orthodontics today, does its work in a much shorter period of time. This type of appliance is attached directly to the teeth with braces, which places undue pressure on the teeth and can create some undesirable consequences. It is my opinion, therefore, that its use should be avoided. (Dentists, please see the entry in Appendix C on epigenetic orthodontics, which goes into the scientific rationale for this type of treatment and why RPE should not be used.) Unfortunately, many traditional orthodontists still use this technique in combination with surgery to achieve their goals. I am of the strong belief that slow palatal expansion with FFO works much better to obtain a more stable correction of the upper jaw without the undesirable side effects of RPE or surgery.

THE MIDPALATAL SUTURE PRINCIPLE

There is a biological fact that allows FFO to be so effective. The midpalatal suture is located in the center of the roof of the mouth. It is a fibrous connection between the two bones that form the roof of the mouth. A key principle to understand—and one that traditional dentistry has not yet recognized—is that this suture remains viable and living all throughout life and therefore permits significant expansion of the upper jaw at any stage of life. This fact allows for the general enlargement of existing bone structure that can occur with FFO appliances.

Dentists and orthodontists, myself included, were incorrectly taught in dental school that this midpalatal suture calcifies over and that the two adjacent bones become fused together at around ages twelve to fourteen. Unless they have been enlightened, dentists may still believe that surgery is necessary to widen the upper jaw on teens and adults alike.

Unfortunately, for millions of patients treated over many decades, unnecessary surgeries have been performed because of this belief. The theory that the midpalatal suture calcifies has been proven wrong by the successful expansion of the upper jaws on thousands of adults without surgery, including many patients well into their seventies. Note the dramatic change in the before and after pictures shown below taken of a patient in her late thirties who was treated with FFO and braces—without extractions or surgery.

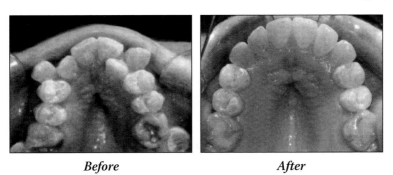

Before   *After*

MUSCLE ADAPTATION TAKES TIME

Another important concept to understand is that while the bone structures are being changed in size and position, another phenomenon is occurring simultaneously. The muscles responsible for the jaw movements have to accommodate the new positions of the bone structures. An important biological principle to understand is "teeth dominate, muscles and joints accommodate." In simple terms, this means that when a person bites down, the muscles move to direct the jaw (which has highly flexible joints) to where the teeth fit together most comfortably. When changing the position of the lower jaw, the muscles will also need time to adjust to a new position. The muscles have been previously programmed to contract and relax in a certain way, so to deprogram them and to have them act differently takes time. This phenomenon of gradual muscle accommodation is the body's protective mechanism so that muscles do not become uncoordinated with the many movements required for normal living.

This speaks to another advantage to the slow expansion process: The muscles and bone structures need to be allowed to change in concert with each other. There is another positive effect that occurs when expanding the upper jaw. When you consider that the bone at the roof of the mouth is the same bone at the floor of the nasal passageway, widening the palate of the mouth will widen the nasal passages as well. This creates a better ability for a patient to breathe through his or her nose, which is a great benefit for a person with a sleep disorder, as explained in Chapter 5.

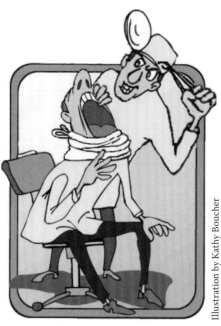

Illustration by Kathy Boucher

"Orthodontics does not have to be as painful as pulling teeth."

EXTRACTION OF PERMANENT TEETH NOT NEEDED!

As discussed previously, and thanks to Dr. Tweed's input, the traditional orthodontic approach to correcting crowded teeth in narrow jaws has been the removal of up to four permanent teeth. The need for extraction of permanent teeth is virtually eliminated, however, by using FFO. (Wisdom teeth, also known as third molars, are the notable exception.)

Crowded teeth are almost always the result of narrow jaw structures, not teeth that are too big. Larger teeth are actually an advantage when it comes to creating a full, beautiful smile because the arch form can be enlarged in order to create the space needed for those teeth. The FFO method eliminates the narrowness of the jaws and the crowding without the removal of any permanent teeth. It also is a very positive step toward preventing overbites, potential TMJ problems, and future problems with obstructive sleep apnea.

One of the more common reasons for extracting permanent teeth is the presence of an overbite. Traditional orthodontists may remove two teeth on the upper dental arch in order to pull the front teeth back to match the lower teeth. As you will see in my explanations in the next section, the extraction of teeth on the upper arch is a big mistake since it does nothing to address the fact that the lower jaw is trapped behind the upper front teeth. This can lead to substantial TMJ dysfunctions later in life. From an aesthetic standpoint, the avoidance of extractions gives the face a full and balanced facial profile.

With all that said, I believe that the wisdom of the old axiom "never say never" comes into play here. There are three notable exceptions to nonextraction treatment. The first is when extreme protrusion of the front teeth is present. Typically, this protrusion is the result of a skeletal deficiency, which is a result of growth patterns altered by undesirable oral habits (especially mouth breathing). However, the determination whether to extract teeth or not is made after the expansion with FFO (to be discussed in Key #1) has given the patient the full arch form necessary to make that decision. The second exception is when a patient cannot be motivated to follow the prescribed wear and activation necessary. Lastly, if the improvements in the arch form from the use of a fixed expansion appliance (because of a cooperation problem) do not create enough room to accommodate all the permanent teeth, extractions then may become necessary.

"Nothing is as powerful as an idea whose time has come."
—Victor Hugo

PART II

THE LAUSON SYSTEM: NINE KEYS TO LOWER FACIAL HARMONY

*"Once we rid ourselves of traditional thinking,
we can get on with creating the future."*
—James Bertrand

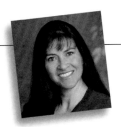

As demonstrated by over five thousand successful cases treated over a twenty-five year period, Functional Facial Orthopedics, combined with braces or Invisalign, can solve almost all dental occlusion (bite) and lower facial harmony problems, without the use of either surgery or removal of permanent teeth. With braces or Invisalign alone, it is not possible to routinely achieve the objectives laid out in The Lauson System.

Nine keys have been laid out in a logical order for you to follow. I have listed the keys in the order of their importance, considering the health and appearance of the total person. However, it is important to know that the first six keys are not widely recognized as important by many traditionalists. In fact, many in the dental community do not realize the fundamental importance of these keys and their relationship to orthodontic treatment. However, keys seven through nine are widely recognized as important by all orthodontists.

These keys all tend to build upon each other as orthodontics is performed, and without meeting the objective of a foundational key, the remaining keys are much more difficult, or impossible, to achieve. For instance, if the upper jaw is narrow and a correction is not made to make a more fully developed arch form (Key #1), then unobstructed nasal breathing (Key #2) and proper forward positioning of the lower jaw (Key #3) will be more difficult to achieve. In addition to that, healthy TMJ function (Key #4) could be compromised, and ideal head posture (Key #5) may be negatively affected. You get the idea. As you can see, the importance of each key and how it impacts the other keys is imperative to understand so that the best possible results can be achieved. The functions of different parts of our bodies all work in conjunction with each other.

We are meant to be whole and complete human beings. The Lauson System helps us to be that way.

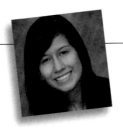

CHAPTER 4

Key #1: Fully Developed Upper Jaw

The word maxilla is the medical name for the part of the anatomy we commonly call the upper jaw. The upper jaw forms the roof of the mouth and is the frame around which the upper teeth are held. The upper jaw also contains the nasal passageway since the same bone that is the roof of the mouth is also the bone that forms the floor of the nasal passageway. A narrow upper jaw is the biggest culprit and the cause of most orthodontic problems.

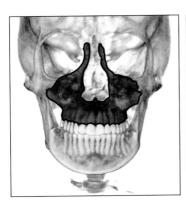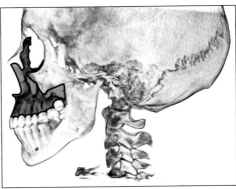

As is evident by the majority of patients who pass through my office, a narrow or underdeveloped maxilla is the root of almost all orthodontic problems. I have included a review in Appendix C that finds that 95% of the patients in the author's orthodontic practice have a deficient maxilla. This statistic is based in the patient load and not in the general population. It does certainly raise a red flag that orthodontists need to really evaluate whether the maxilla is an ideal shape and size in each patient. Also in the appendix is an article, "A New Gold Standard for Orthodontic Evaluations," which includes a reference to the need for this evaluation.

The main concern regarding this narrow maxillary condition is insufficient bone structure to support the size of the naturally occurring teeth. In other words, the upper jaw is just too small for all the teeth. This forces the teeth out of proper alignment and is a setup for many maladies inside the mouth, such as uneven wear of tooth enamel and bone, gum recession, and oral hygiene issues. These problems are seemingly small, but can lead to larger issues discussed later in this book. An underdeveloped maxilla can lead to a receded or weak chin because the narrow upper jaw can cause a restrictive trapping of the lower jaw in its growth stage (explained further in Chapter 6). "Buck teeth"—a phenomenon seen when the upper teeth are forced too far forward—can also result. A narrow upper jaw also causes reduction to the nasal breathing capacity, which in severe cases can result in a mouth-breathing habit with many undesired effects. In short, the maxilla is a ground-zero source for many health issues.

"Education consists mainly of what we have unlearned."
—Mark Twain

Traditional orthodontics has long recognized the narrow upper jaw as a major cause of misaligned teeth; however, it still sometimes calls for the maxilla to be left in a narrow state as long as the condition hasn't caused a crossbite (when the upper teeth are positioned inside the lower teeth).

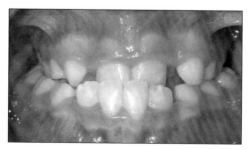

This picture shows an example of a crossbite,
both in the front and back teeth.

Traditional orthodontists may solve the problem of the crowded and misaligned teeth by extracting as many as four permanent teeth. In some cases, however, they may suggest to accomplish the widening with a surgical procedure. Sally's case, discussed in Chapter 2, is a prime example of a case in which extractions are more commonly prescribed to eliminate crowding.

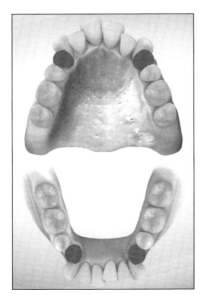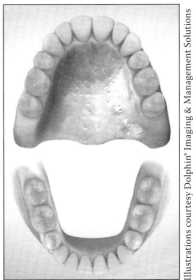

Extraction treatment shown

In the pictures above, the first picture shows the teeth marked that would be extracted and the second picture shows the result after closure of the space with braces. The teeth are straight, but the narrowness remains. This result is considered perfectly acceptable for the traditional orthodontist, but leaves the arch forms narrow and can cause many future problems, not the least of which is the narrowness of the smile. For those who are widely concerned with their looks, a well-developed upper jaw creates strong, balanced facial contours and the potential for an unforgettable smile. Consider the parade of cover girls you have seen or the "movie star smile" exemplified by the picture below of the famous actress Julia Roberts. Although she was not a patient of mine, her beautiful smile is a great example of the full, ideally developed maxilla.

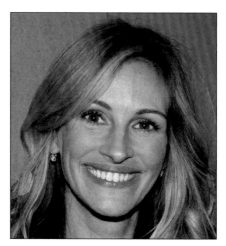

Actress Julia Roberts

From an aesthetic standpoint, the underdeveloped maxilla can cause what cosmetic dentists call "dark triangles." These are dark, shadowy, triangular-shaped spaces between one's teeth and at the widest corner of one's smile, as indicated by the arrows on the picture below. The teeth look set in from the rest of the mouth and may even give a person a "sunken cheeks" look. These dark triangles indicate that the dental arch form is constricted, causing the front teeth to be accentuated or to appear too large. Many times this is the result of leaving the arch form constricted; no "movie star smile" is achieved, and the dreaded dark triangles remain!

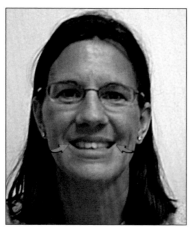
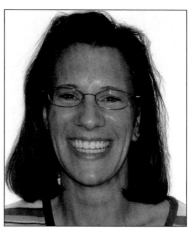

Before FFO: Dark Triangles   *After FFO: No Dark Triangles*

Genetics, bad habits, and perhaps a little bad luck can cause the maxilla to develop improperly. A narrow maxilla is also implicated in a host of other issues: poor chewing, gum disease, sinus conditions, TMD neck pain, and eye and ear problems. A narrow upper jaw can cause nasal obstruction, which can lead to mouth breathing, a condition that causes a host of problems all its own. Having an upper jaw that is an ideal size and shape is closely tied to a person's ability to breathe properly through his or her nose. After their maxillas were widened, many of my patients who suffered with asthma felt profound relief with their breathing problems.

THE MAXILLA HAS THE POWER TO SHAPE ONE'S QUALITY OF LIFE!

Amazingly, if a narrow upper jaw is left uncorrected, a person's entire posture can be affected. Here's how this condition can develop: To compensate for a narrow upper jaw, a person must bring his or her lower jaw back too far in order to get the teeth to come together to chew. This in turn causes the head to move forward unnaturally. While seemingly a subtle gesture, over time it can affect the entire neck and spinal system. Over time, this fundamentally unnatural forward head posture forces the rest of the body to also alter itself. Eventually, the entire body can become out of alignment, resulting in a stooped, bent-over stance as one ages. By correcting the maxilla early, the mouth and jaws are brought into alignment, and the head is carried in its normal position, allowing good body posture to follow along. For further detail on how this condition develops, see Chapter 8.

Another cause of an improperly developed upper arch form is the presence of adverse oral habits. Thumb or finger sucking as a child, nail biting, and pushing the tongue against the front teeth (tongue thrust) can all have a negative impact on the growth of the maxilla. Over time, these seemingly harmless habits can create destructive pressure on the teeth and supporting bone structures. These habits are fully addressed in Chapter 9.

SOLVING THE PROBLEM:
THE LAUSON SYSTEM SOLUTION

Although having a narrow upper jaw is a common problem, it is a treatable one. The maxilla can be safely and gently expanded over time, leading to an ideal arch form. It is preferable that this procedure be done at an early stage in a person's life since a normal growth pattern can be established at that time. However, as you will see, this expansion of the upper jaw can be done at any age—without surgery.

The Lauson System is based on one important fact: The midpalatal suture (the connection of the two halves of the upper jaw at the roof of the mouth) remains viable throughout life, allowing the upper jaw to be gradually widened at any age without surgery. In fact, it has been shown that stem cells, which have the capacity to form new bone, exist within the sutures and are always ready to spring into action when properly stimulated.

Traditional teaching of orthodontics states that after about the age of twelve, the midpalatal suture fuses, preventing the upper jaw from being altered without surgery. This actually is not true. The book review of *Epigenetic Orthodontics in Adults* and review of the medical field of craniosacral therapy, found in Appendix C, give more scientific evidence for this truth. Once this is understood and accepted, a whole new world of opportunity will be opened up. The more conservative FFO treatment eliminates teeth extractions and/or surgical risks. Down the road, the potential, unintended consequences of surgery can be poor healing or a poor fit of the reconstructed upper jaw, and since the removal of several permanent teeth is a common practice of traditional orthodontics, this leaves smaller jaws and can contribute to overall instability.

Successful treatment with FFO has proven that teeth extraction is virtually unnecessary. The Lauson System can result in a properly sized maxilla for patients of all ages, even those well into their "golden years," by using customized, removable appliances.

"If it has been done before, it is probably possible."

—Anonymous

Occasionally, a parent may be concerned about changes in facial appearance when considering FFO treatment. The motherly, loving, untrained eye may think little Mary looks just fine. "We don't want our daughter to look funny!" is an occasional response. However, a parent quickly gains confidence when shown before and after photos of previously treated patients. "They look beautiful!" is the standard comment made by the parent. Yes, the power of the maxilla to redefine the face is truly remarkable!

The following case study is a good example of the use of FFO to expand the maxilla to an ideal shape to create a handsome, movie star smile.

Rob was sixteen years old when he came to my office with substantial crowding of his front teeth. His upper jaw was narrower than what is considered ideal, and his lower teeth were leaning inward toward his tongue, a commonly seen situation in any orthodontic office. Conventional orthodontics typically would have recommended the removal of four first bicuspid teeth and then the straightening of the remaining teeth with braces.

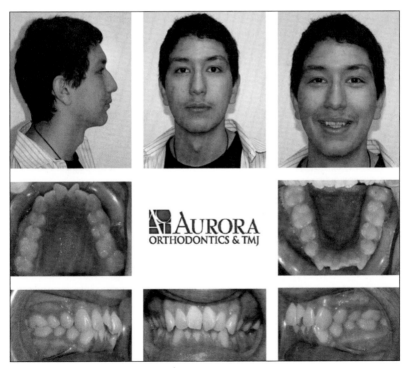

Pretreatment photos showing crowding and narrow arches

Instead, we widened both the upper and lower dental arches using Schwarz expansion appliances, which took about four months. Then we placed braces to finish his treatment in just under two years of overall treatment time. This ended up being a straightforward case with a beautiful, nonextraction result. Note that in the before pictures, the corners of Rob's smile showed dark triangles at the sides of his teeth, due to constriction of the upper dental arch. After treatment, the dark triangles were all filled in with teeth.

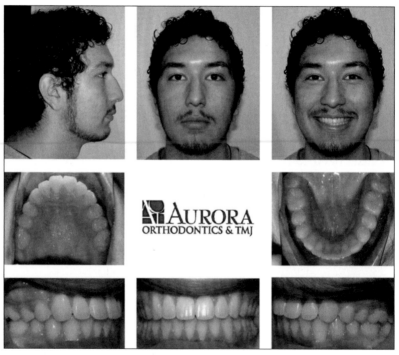

Photos at completion of treatment

After treatment was completed, Rob's smile was full and confident. This result would not have been possible without the expansion of the arch forms. It is commonly believed that maxillofacial surgery is necessary (after twelve to fourteen years of age) to widen the bones of the maxilla to achieve the desired result. Extraction of permanent teeth to reduce crowding would be another choice; however, this leaves the patient with less teeth and arches that are still too narrow. As you can see, The Lauson System can accomplish a beautiful, stable result without invasive procedures.

36

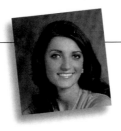

CHAPTER 5

Key #2: Unobstructed Nasal Breathing

T his key is among the first discussed for an important reason. A person's ability to breathe properly through his or her nose, without obstruction, is critical to his or her health and vitality in many ways; it cannot be overemphasized as a health or quality-of-life issue. Obstructions, whatever their cause, need to be evaluated and eliminated. Period! Without the elimination of the obstruction, mouth breathing can result and lead to many avoidable problems, including poor facial and dental development.

It is important to recognize that, although it is recommended that a child be evaluated by an orthodontist by age seven, the astute parent or the child's doctor or dentist can recognize many of the problems associated with airway obstruction much before that age. Perhaps the most obvious of these problems is when a baby or very young child makes excessive noise while breathing during either waking or sleeping hours. This is a sign that there could be an obstructed nasal passageway present that needs to be evaluated. This problem, at whatever age it's detected, is entirely treatable and must be addressed.

WHAT IS THE REAL PROBLEM?

One memorable February day, a mother brought in her cherubic, seven-year-old son to my office on the recommendation of their family dentist. After just one glance at the dry, chapped lips of my new, young patient, I could tell that Brett (as we'll call him) was developing a potentially serious problem. His mom wasn't particularly concerned about her son's dry lips, but she had noticed a number of other symptoms that worried her. This is a classic example of the opportunity an orthodontist has to pick up on the problem of airway obstruction.

"Brett always seems to be waking up with a sore throat and a stuffy nose," she fretted. "And in the last few years he's been listless and always looks like he is really tired out. Lately, he can barely force himself to get through the day."

He did indeed look tired and worn out—he should have been brimming with all the vitality one expects from a seven-year-old. After I had been observing Brett for merely a few minutes, I felt confident that I had answers—and hope—for his worried mother. All of those clues were classic symptoms of the condition known as nasopharyngeal obstruction (NPO). The little guy was a mouth breather!

Mouth breathing sounds deceptively mundane and inconsequential as a diagnosis goes; however, it can be both a cause and an effect of serious structural and physiological changes in one's mouth and nasal passageway. It can initiate a complex chain of events that, over time, can even significantly change one's appearance and health for the worse.

THE DANGERS OF MOUTH BREATHING

In simple terms, oxygen is the body's number-one nutrient, and a person will die when deprived of it for even a few minutes. Because of this, the body has a built-in protection mechanism. When oxygen can't effectively be drawn in through the nose, the body moves to plan B and draws it in through the mouth. For all intents and purposes, that would seem to solve the problem, except there's a catch: the body isn't meant to breathe through the mouth except in an emergency situation requiring a high level of oxygen, such as in athletics.

When a person breathes through his or her mouth in a normal, everyday, nonstressful situation, the body's knee-jerk solution triggers an avalanche of unintended consequences. Left unchecked, these consequences ripple outward to include more and more conditions and disorders that can impact one's health well into adulthood. All in all, I consider NPO possibly the most devastating, but absolutely preventable, facial development problem for a youngster. It's almost impossible to overemphasize how important it is to correct this condition at as young an age as possible.

Consider all the ways in which Brett's health was impacted by this deceptively simple problem. When Brett became a mouth breather, he opened the door to throat irritations (including bacteria and viruses)—all of which the naturally occurring mucus in the nose is designed to capture. What's more, the act of open-mouthed breathing itself alters the proper placement of the tongue. With the mouth open, the lower jaw is lower, pulling the tongue away from its proper placement, which is up against the roof of the mouth. The dropped posture of the tongue and the subsequent understimulation to the upper jaw leads to the underdevelopment (or narrowing) of the upper arch. This narrowing of the upper jaw (see Chapter 4) leads to the trapping effect of the lower jaw (see Chapter 6) by putting it into a retruded position, meaning it is set too far back in the face. This also leads to other adverse consequences: that of the head going into a forward posture (which is discussed in more detail in Chapter 8) and a later-in-life, serious condition known as obstructive sleep apnea (details in Chapter 9). Childhood, when bones are still growing, is the best time to correct NPO and an underdeveloped upper jaw so that normal growth and development can occur from that point forward.

I knew that dry air flowing over his teeth would inflame Brett's gums, so after observing his dry, parted lips, the presence of gum redness and swelling was no surprise to me. Brett had been told to brush his teeth better by the family dental hygienist, who may not have told him that the inflamed gums were a result of the boy's mouth-breathing habit. Because a dry mouth also dries up saliva, the body's natural decay-preventative substance, tooth decay was also likely. Even Brett's listlessness could be traced to mouth breathing. When the nose is obstructed, the body's plan B may attempt to get the job done, but the fact remains: Oxygen doesn't reach the body as efficiently when breathing through the mouth.

If left uncorrected, Brett's mouth breathing would lay a trap for a very dangerous future: the debilitating condition called obstructive sleep apnea (OSA), wherein a sleeping person momentarily stops breathing multiple times throughout the night. Although a child can have it, OSA usually doesn't develop until adulthood. Unless the nasal obstruction is addressed when the patient is a child, it begins to lay the groundwork for OSA, as well as many other conditions. This very important topic of OSA will be discussed more in depth in Chapter 9.

Other suspected relationships link NPO as a cause for sudden infant death syndrome (SIDS) and attention deficit disorder (ADD and ADHD). I have included a reference in the appendix from WebMD.com, which goes into more detail about how NPO can cause these types of problems. It points out how critical it is to make these corrections in a youngster's life. It continues to amaze me how very important a normal nasal breathing pattern is. All these NPO problems begin early, so there's no time to waste.

In short, NPO and mouth breathing are vexing conditions with many ramifications. In my opinion, no other single, preventable dysfunction in the human body has quite the same multiple, wide-ranging causes and effects. No matter how the nasal obstruction develops, the outcome can be devastating for a young child, as the flow chart shown in the appendix fully explains. The good news is nasal obstruction and mouth breathing can be prevented or corrected. So now let's begin to wrestle down the causes of this deceptively simple condition.

WHAT CAUSES NASAL OBSTRUCTIONS?

As we've seen, obstructions of the nasal passageway create a domino effect and impact the entire health of the patient. What are the common causes of NPO?

ALLERGIC RHINITIS

A very common cause of NPO is an obstruction produced by allergies (allergic rhinitis). Inflammation caused by the presence of an allergen results in swelling of the mucus membranes on the inside of the nasal passageways. This swelling reduces the opening of the nasal passageway, potentially causing an obstruction leading to mere nasal stuffiness or mouth breathing.

Nasal sprays and lavages (nasal irrigation therapy in which mucus and debris are flushed from the nose and sinuses) can help, but if the condition is severe, an evaluation should be completed by a physician whose specialty is working with allergies. Other causes include cysts, polyps, and tumors. These should be ruled out with an evaluation by an otolaryngologist, a physician specializing in diseases of the ear, nose, and throat.

DEVIATED SEPTUM

The medical term deviated septum has entered our general vernacular courtesy of palookas whose schnozzolas got busted in the boxing arena and would-be-beautiful people who weren't happy with the nose God gave them. The deviation is sometimes genetic, or it can occur during childbirth, in a childhood football game, or in a car accident. The condition results when the septum, which consists of the bone and cartilage separating the nose into two nostrils, deviates from one side to the other. Whatever its cause, a deviated septum should not be taken lightly. It can be a serious condition and is a common cause of nasal obstruction and mouth breathing.

A deviated septum is exceptionally common in people with narrow upper jaws. To better understand this condition, imagine a box. A cardboard strip—that's the nasal septum—divides the box. When the upper jaw (the box) doesn't grow to its normal size, pressure is exerted on the inside, and that center strip of cardboard (septum) tends to bend and get smashed down. As it's displaced, it bunches either to the left or to the right, causing the cardboard (septum) to deviate.

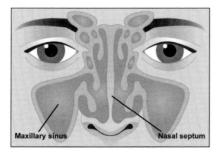 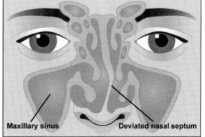

Illustration by Todd Gilmore

Normal   *Abnormal*

In a person with a deviated septum, the smashed center strip in the nose may block normal breathing function. Again, the person resorts to the one open highway left for air, the mouth. The medical community of specialists in otolaryngology will frequently recommend surgery to eliminate a deviated septum.

It is my belief that a deviated septum is almost always the result of poor development of the upper jaw and not a separate development problem itself. By widening the upper jaw to an ideal dimension, I have eliminated this deviated septum problem, which causes nasal obstruction, on many patients. When the upper jaw is allowed to expand, the septum may straighten on its own. Therefore, I always ask my patients with deviated septums to hold off on nasal surgery until after we expand the upper jaw. They seem pleased at the prospect of avoiding this unpleasant surgery, and after we complete the expansion, the surgery is rarely needed. To see the gradual but inexorable process take place—the body, in effect, healing itself—is a beautiful thing to behold, not unlike a flower finally going into full bloom.

TONSILS AND ADENOIDS

Tonsils are those little sacs that you can see hanging at the back of the throat, and adenoids are hidden above the tonsils. They both are sacs of lymphatic tissue, which are the first scrubbing filters against the bacteria and viruses that enter the mouth and nasal passages. In function, they're akin to the lymph glands lying astride the sides of the neck, as well as in the groin and armpits. The difference is, while the other glands remain vigilant for a lifetime, tonsils and adenoids tend to outgrow their usefulness as a person gets older.

When I was a child in the 1950s, almost everyone had their tonsils removed, as did I, at age two. For several decades, tonsillectomies were part of accepted medical wisdom, whether the tonsils were infected or not. It went from being a surgical procedure to almost a rite of passage, becoming nearly as routine as losing one's baby teeth.

Eventually it was debated whether or not it was appropriate to routinely remove tonsils. The concern was that the procedure removed lymphatic tissue, which could compromise the immune system. (This was later disproved;

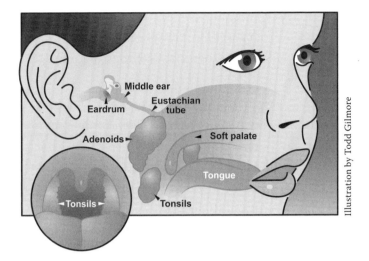

those who have large tonsils and adenoids also have plenty of lymphatic tissue in other areas.) Inevitably, this caused the pendulum to swing the other way and for several decades almost no one had them removed at all.

As for adenoids, they may lack the legendary star power of the tonsils, but when it comes to childhood torments, they have their own important role to play. First of all, you can't see the adenoids because they're hidden above and behind the prominently visible tonsils. But adenoids still behave like the proverbial eight-hundred-pound gorilla when it comes to significant mouth, nose, and ear problems. Enlarged adenoids are a main culprit of severe childhood earaches. If a child suffers from persistent pain inside the ear, it's a red-flag warning to look for enlarged adenoids. When they become oversized, adenoids encroach on the Eustachian tube, the conduit to the middle ear that regulates ear pressure and balance. But like an oversized pillow taking up space, when the adenoids are swollen they tend to impinge on the Eustachian tube. In effect, this allows bacteria to puddle up in the tube, and from there the bacteria back up into the middle ear, causing painful infections.

Today, many family physicians and pediatricians still resist removal of tonsils and adenoids, and most doctors use a formula to decide when that should happen: If three or more infection episodes occur in a twelve-month period, approval for removal is granted. Chronically inflamed tonsils are a breeding ground for colds, hoarseness, bad breath, and constant sore throat miseries, including strep throat. However, there is little consideration given to the possible disorders caused by the enlarged tonsils or adenoids. These disorders, such as NPO, cause mouth breathing and poor growth of the facial structures.

Otolaryngology specialists typically recognize that there are other very legitimate reasons for having tonsils and adenoids removed other than the three-infection rule. I find that these well-informed otolaryngologists are a pleasure to work with because they are more aware that NPO can cause significant facial developmental problems, and they readily see the need to remove obstructive tonsils and adenoids.

MOUTH BREATHING AND ITS EFFECTS, ESPECIALLY ON CHILDREN

It is extremely important to identify and correct nasal obstruction and mouth breathing during childhood. If solved then, a youngster is saved from years of difficulties ranging from abnormal growth of the mouth and facial structures to an array of painful conditions and even disease. But because the effects of mouth breathing are so subtle and incremental, years can be lost before the effects of the problem are recognized. Sometimes people don't understand why mouth breathing is cause for alarm. Other times, they aren't even aware it's happening. When I informed one mom and dad that their eight-year-old child was a mouth breather, they were incredulous. The child's mouth appeared closed, but was indeed slightly open. When I had them observe this, along with the dry, chapped lips, they realized the impact.

People tend to think of mouth breathing as something a person does when they've participated in an athletic event, such as climbing the summit of one of Colorado's 14,000-foot mountain peaks—the mouth is open wide and the person is sucking in air with deep breaths. But chronic mouth breathing is a very different thing, often marked by only the very slightest parting of the lips.

To understand the unintended consequences of mouth breathing, an explanation of normal, healthy air exchange is in order. Normal nasal breathing affects airflow into the body by warming and moistening the air. This actually prepares the air for the lungs so they can perform their normal oxygen exchange. Studies have shown that mouth breathers exchange oxygen as much as 40% less effectively than normal nasal breathers. Since oxygen is the body's number-one nutrient, depriving it of the required oxygen level has all sorts of negative consequences, including possible death.

But how would mouth breathing contribute to listlessness? When it comes to the serious effects of nasal obstruction and mouth breathing, this may be the most fascinating, unintended consequence of all. The inefficient absorption of oxygen in the human body is why mouth breathers typically are marked by a dull and apathetic look. They may not do well in school and seem not fully engaged in what's happening around them. Some tend to withdraw, to become antisocial, and typically stay away from sports. Sometimes mouth breathers are stereotyped as slow or unintelligent. But their natural intelligence is not to blame; they're basically suffering from chronic apoxia—oxygen deprivation.

In fact, recent studies have linked airway obstructions to the very common childhood problem of ADHD. One study showed that among ADHD children, who also had excessively large tonsils, once the tonsils were removed, the ADHD was eliminated in over 50% of those in the study. (Please refer to the appendix to the chart on NPO for a more thorough look at this serious problem.) If there is any debate between the efficacies of nose breathing versus mouth breathing, this chart should settle it.

One of the most gratifying parts of being an orthodontist is to be able to diagnose and treat these subtle, but profound, effects that have such an impact well into adulthood. It brings me great delight to confront the presence and the cause of these airway obstructions and motivate parents, patients, and other doctors to take them seriously.

Yet, when I point out these serious effects of mouth breathing to parents, the reaction is often disbelief. Then, a little later, as they've had a chance to absorb the idea, they look as if the weight of the world has been lifted off their shoulders. There's nothing more troubling than seeing a delightful youngster slowly start morphing into a sickly child. If an obstructed nasal passageway, resulting in mouth breathing, is missed as the cause of these problems, families often resort to years of trial-and-error solutions, treating the child with everything from children's vitamins to drug prescriptions (and later in life, medical procedures and surgeries), which could have been avoided.

The story of the following patient illustrates this very important concept. When I first saw Karen, six months shy of her twelfth birthday, she had substantial teeth crowding (especially on the lower jaw), an excessive overbite, and was a mouth breather. She also had skeletal Class II relationships (see Chapter 12 for classifications), and the molars were in crossbite on the right side. Both arches were substantially constricted, but the crossbite was an indication that the upper arch was more constricted than the lower. This constriction caused the lower jaw to be trapped behind the upper and was already having an effect on her jaw joints, as she couldn't open her lower jaw in a normal fashion (Chapters 6 and 7 will discuss these problems in more depth).

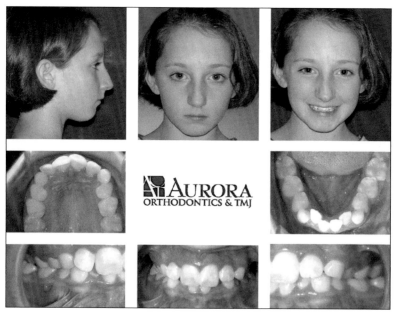

Pretreatment photos

Karen also had a loss of the normal curvature of her neck, as seen below in the x-ray taken at her initial exam. This x-ray also showed enlarged adenoid tissue, which her otolaryngologist removed following our treatment recommendation to eliminate upper-airway obstruction.

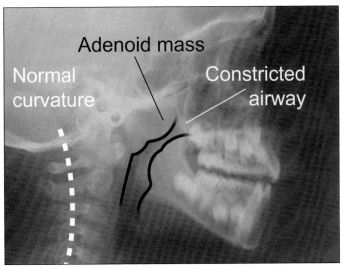

Cephalometric x-ray taken before treatment shows a loss of the normal curvature of the neck and enlargement of the adenoids

In our initial phase, we treated Karen with an upper Schwarz appliance with an anterior bite plate and a lower Schwarz appliance (see Appendix A for description of all treatment appliances). While expanding both the upper and lower jaws, the bite plate helped to correct the deep bite and freed up the trapped lower jaw, allowing it to move forward into a more desirable position so that the jaw joints could operate normally. Once this was accomplished, Karen was instructed to wear the appliances at night-time only until her permanent teeth came in. With proper breathing and function restored, this became a routine case and was completed with eighteen months of braces.

All the goals of the nine keys to lower facial harmony were achieved with this treatment protocol. Had the initial orthopedic phase not been completed and the ideal nasal breathing restored, the likely treatment plan would have included the removal of permanent teeth, leaving the dental arches constricted and possibly increasing the TMJ dysfunction. This also would have left the lower jaw trapped in a retruded position, further accentuating Karen's nose in an unflattering way. Although Karen still has a slightly recessed lower jaw, her profile was improved and resulted in a great smile, and her TMJ and bite are now in harmony.

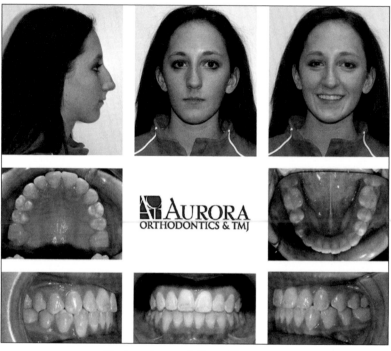

Photos at completion of treatment

In conclusion, mouth breathing is an important indicator of overall health; it should be taken very seriously and a solution should be found early. The impact that an orthodontist can have on the future health of a patient is profound. The Lauson System detects and treats these airway concerns, which are instrumental in prevention of obstructive sleep apnea later in life. Chapter 9 explores this topic in more depth, but parents should take heart that a solution can virtually always be found.

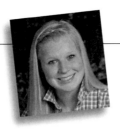

CHAPTER 6

Key #3: Proper Forward Positioning of Lower Jaw

A key factor to lower facial harmony is for the lower jaw to be in balance with the fully developed upper jaw (Key #1). When this occurs, the facial balance that results gives a person a most attractive and healthy relationship. This allows the adult woman to enjoy a confident and attractive profile that gives proper support to her lips and creates a natural fullness. Desire for this look has created a Botox explosion in plastic surgeon's offices. A properly placed lower jaw, complementing this fully developed upper jaw, creates the gentleman's ideal profile and gives him an air of strength and trustworthiness.

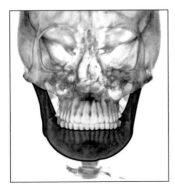
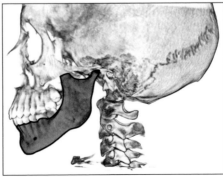

This, of course, is the desire of any parent for his or her developing child and should be one of the objectives of any treatment plan. However, this result does not automatically happen, nor is it the result of the more traditional orthodontic treatment methods. If either the upper jaw or the lower jaw ends up being underdeveloped, then the compromised profile will have a negative impact on the person's psyche and his or her overall health.

One of the most important concepts to understand is how lower facial harmonies develop (or fail to develop). For the face to develop in a healthy and well-balanced fashion, the order in which the upper and lower jaws develop is extremely important. As stated in Chapter 4, the upper jaw must be expanded to a full arch form, allowing the lower jaw to develop to its normal size, shape, and position. It stands to reason that if the upper jaw is constricted, the lower jaw will also be restricted in its development and placement.

TRAPPING OF THE LOWER JAW

One of the most common problems that can occur in facial development is the trapping of the lower jaw to restrict its forward development. This leads to overbites and other development problems. To understand how this can happen, let's go back to a very early stage in a child's development.

When looking at a newborn baby, it is noticeable that he or she has virtually no chin—and not just because of baby fat. The reality is that the newborn actually has more development in the midface area, consequently giving the baby a very round-faced look. As the baby matures into childhood, the lower jaw and chin begin to emerge. More growth in the lower jaw occurs as it moves downward and forward. Between the ages of six and eight, the permanent front teeth emerge into the mouth. If there is an ideal facial-growth pattern established, the teeth begin to match as they should when they enter the mouth.

Very commonly, however, the midface development at ages six to eight is still significantly forward of the lower jaw in its development. When this occurs, overbites can develop because the upper front teeth may come in too fast and too far, causing the lower teeth and jaw to come in behind them so that the lower jaw is trapped into a retruded position. In addition to being caused by an excessive overbite, this trapping can also be the result of an underdeveloped or narrow upper jaw, as shown in the pictures below. The connection between the normal, fully developing maxilla and its effect on normal growth and positioning of the mandible is evident. Enlarged tonsils and adenoids that create a mouth-breathing habit, or even an adverse oral habit, such as finger or thumb sucking, can also cause this trapping effect and set the lower jaw up to function improperly.

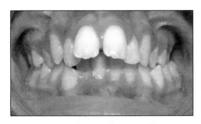 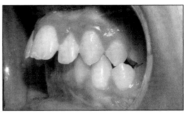

These photos illustrate an example of a narrow upper jaw causing a trapping of the lower teeth and jaw.

The trapping of the lower jaw doesn't cause a lack of growth of the lower jaw so much as an actual posterior displacement of the entire jaw. This has huge implications and is a primary factor in the resulting TMJ dysfunctions so common among people with retruded lower jaws. Suffice it to say that it is very important to "untrap," or free up, a lower jaw for development at an early age to allow it to catch up with upper jaw growth and ultimately balance with the fully developed upper jaw.

Another less common condition is when the upper jaw becomes trapped behind the lower jaw, creating an underbite. This happens when the lower jaw develops ahead of the upper jaw. Upper-airway obstructions early in life can be major contributing causes of this condition as the limited air intake creates a need for mouth breathing, which in turn causes a lower-tongue posture and a lack of stimulation of the upper jaw's development. This type of functional problem also needs early correction. Many times a frustrated parent is told by his or her dentist or orthodontist that the child will have to wait until he or she is at least sixteen years of age to have surgery to set back the prominent lower jaw.

This has been a traditional approach for many years. The good news is that with the use of FFO, these skeletal bone structures of the face can be corrected at any age because, as explained in Chapter 4, the human skull has viable sutures that allow for the expansion of the bone structure at any time.

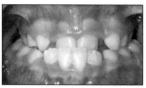 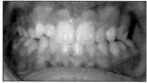 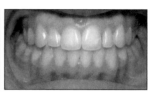

Before Treatment   *After Expansion*   *After Final Treatment*

Whereas underdevelopment can be handled with these orthopedic procedures, the surgical procedure has a much more difficult time adding new bone. Surgeons are much better at taking away excess bone, so it stands to reason that they might approach these skeletal problems from a different perspective than the dental professional using FFO. Key #4 (Healthy TMJ Function) points out that a great deal of inappropriate and unnecessary surgery is performed when surgically lengthening lower jaws to relieve an apparent deficiency or when shortening upper jaws to meet a retruded lower jaw. Either case tends to "lock in" TMJ dysfunction in patients with a posteriorly displaced lower jaw. This surgical procedure creates a far more difficult problem to correct than if it had never been performed in the first place. To avoid mistakes, it is important for the doctor and parent (and patient) to fully understand what the totality of the problem is, including proper TMJ position, before implementing a treatment plan that includes surgery.

SOCIAL IMPLICATIONS

A weak, or retruded, lower jaw has profound social implications and is associated with a passive or weak personality. Right or wrong, a person with a recessed lower jaw is labeled as someone who is severely lacking in self-image and is a pushover when it comes to standing up for himself or herself. Possibly even more importantly, this lower-jaw retrusion can lead to all sorts of unhealthy physical effects, including poor head posture, TMD, and obstructive sleep apnea, which are discussed in forthcoming sections.

Conversely, a person with a protruded lower jaw, like comedian Jay Leno, may appear to look aggressive in nature. Jay has overcome that perception and projects the image of a genuinely nice guy. This lower-jaw protrusion can have such a profound effect on a person's personality that studies have shown that the prison population has a much higher incidence of prominent lower jaws than the population in general. (A side note: Cases of ADHD, a topic discussed in the previous section on NPO, are also predominant within the prison population.) Either way, the solution remains the same: create a healthy relationship between the upper and lower arches with the use of FFO.

FACIAL CLASSIFICATIONS DEFINED

The recessed lower jaw is known among orthodontists as a skeletal Class II relationship. It exists in as much as 40% of the population. The protruded lower jaw is known as a skeletal Class III relationship and exists in about 3-5% of the population. The remaining 50+% of the population are said to have a normal, or Class I, relationship. These relationships also refer to teeth positions that vary from normal (Class I), with upper teeth too far forward (Class II), and lower teeth too far forward (Class III).

Illustrations courtesy Dolphin® Imaging

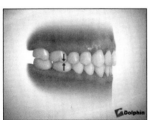 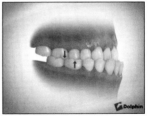

| *Class I* | *Class II* | *Class III* |
| *Normal Relationship* | *Retruded Lower Jaw* | *Protruded Lower Jaw* |

It is fascinating that even though the appearance of a prominent lower jaw exists, almost all of the skeletal Class III relationships are the result of the underdevelopment of the upper jaw, not the overdevelopment of the lower jaw. The prominent lower jaw is mostly an illusion. However, this is not totally accepted in the orthodontic and oral surgery specialties of dentistry. There are still many unnecessary surgeries being performed to move a lower jaw backward to relieve its prominence—all because of a lack of understanding of this relationship and the potential of using FFO to correct an underdeveloped upper jaw.

When eleven-year-old Jake first visited our office with his family, his sister Vanessa was also being evaluated for orthodontic treatment. He didn't have the extreme crowding of teeth that his sister had (she is our Case #8 in Chapter 15), but he did have an extreme overbite (skeletal Class II relationship) and a narrow upper jaw. He also had a chronic mouth-breathing habit, and our evaluation of his tonsils and adenoids revealed a moderate enlargement of each. I did not feel that the size of his tonsils were a major obstacle to Jake gaining a normal, nasal-breathing habit, as tonsils and adenoids normally peak in their size around the age of four and will typically shrink through adolescence.

The treatment plan called for orthopedically widening both jaws and dental arches, which would not only create needed room for all the teeth, but

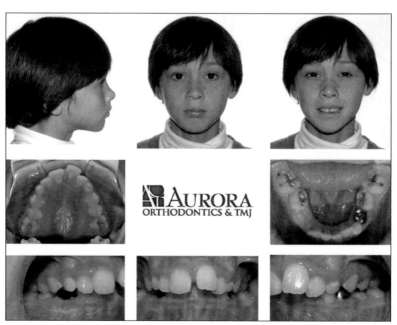

Pretreatment photos showing excessive overbite and narrow dental arches

also provide a better airflow through the nasal passageway. Additionally, the wider upper dental arch would release the lower jaw that was trapped by the narrow upper jaw, allowing it to come forward in a very natural way to correct the overbite and give Jake a much-improved profile. Please note the recessed chin on the before profile photo and compare to the after profile photo.

The treatment began with an upper Schwarz expander, an anterior bite plate, and a lower lip bumper (see Appendix A for description of all treatment appliances). The expansion took about eight months, and we waited about six months afterward for the eruption of permanent teeth to place braces. During this time the mouth breathing stopped and normal nasal breathing was established. With the widening completed and the mouth-breathing habit no longer present, the lower jaw began to move forward naturally, as predicted. Once the remaining permanent teeth came in, we placed braces on Jake's teeth. The braces segment of his treatment was completed in eight months, with the beautiful result seen below. All nine keys of our treatment objectives were achieved.

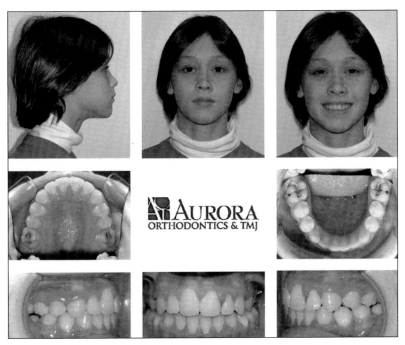

Photos at completion of treatment

I believe that having Jake and his sister, Vanessa, as patients at the same time helped the siblings to motivate each other so that both were able to get great results. Had Jake's treatment been completed with a traditional approach without FFO, he undoubtedly would have had at least two upper permanent bicuspid teeth removed, and possibly even two more on his lower arch. This would have resulted in several undesirable side effects, including the fact that the lower jaw may have remained in a retruded position; this would have been a setup for TMD in future years. Many children have orthodontic treatment started with this type of situation every day. By following the principles of The Lauson System, the unhappy result of future TMJ disorders can be avoided. Now let's investigate further the role of the TMJ.

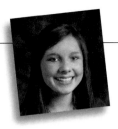

CHAPTER 7

Key #4: Healthy TMJ Function

First of all, what is TMJ, and why would we include information about it in an orthodontic book geared toward treatment of the younger person? Isn't it an affliction for adults to deal with? How do we get it? The following answers may be surprising.

In recent years, the TMJ has become a familiar part of our language. People who suffer from jaw pain commonly say, "I have TMJ." Everybody has a temporomandibular joint, or TMJ—actually two of them, located in front of each ear—which are responsible for allowing the lower jaw to move and for all the wide-ranging motions that are performed effortlessly upon chewing, talking, yawning, laughing, or swallowing. When people have problems with their jaw joint, what they actually mean is that they have TMJ *dysfunction,* or TMD.

The TMJ is especially worthy of attention due to its versatility and functionality. It is important to know that the TMJ is the most complex and active joint in the human body. Composed of only a few ounces of cartilage, bones, ligaments, and muscles, it springs into action as many as one hundred thousand times a day, completing more repetitions than any other similar body part. When functioning properly, it is capable of performing a myriad of intricate maneuvers within seconds, even shifting, when needed, from one dimensional plane to another. But, when it's out of place, it causes considerable pain and discomfort, oftentimes affecting the entire body— causing headaches, ear or vision problems, and even backaches, just to name a few. Because of the TMJ's crucial role in the human body and its intimate connection to the teeth, it is one of the signature components that must be dealt with in respect to any corrections of the mouth, teeth, or jaw.

The following illustration shows the anatomy of the TMJ:

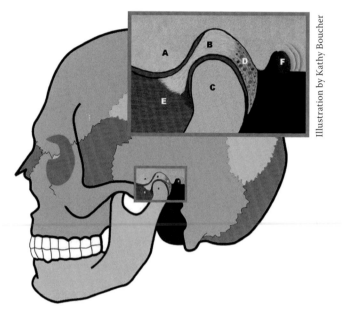

A=Temporal Bone; B=Articular Disc (or just Disc); C=Condyle;
D=Posterior Ligament (containing nerves and blood vessels);
E=Lateral Pterygoid Muscle; F=Ear Canal

So, why talk about the TMJ in a book written about children's ortho-dontics? Simple: The connection of the TMJ to teeth is direct and movement of those teeth affects the TMJs. TMD can start during childhood, when permanent teeth are coming into the mouth. The jaw joints need to be evaluated early so that if a problem exists, it can be corrected during the time that orthodontic treatment is performed. Therefore, an orthodontist or a dentist performing orthodontics should do a thorough evaluation and make a correction if symptoms of TMJ dysfunction begin to develop.

Unfortunately, every dentist performing treatment for TMD sees a great number of patients who previously had orthodontic treatment (and of course many as well who never saw an orthodontist's office) and now are seeking help because of a painful TMJ disorder. They report that the clicking jaws and the problem of the dysfunctional TMJ may or may not have been present, but were not addressed with the patient's original orthodontic treatment. In order to give proper treatment, it becomes necessary to first correct the TMJ problem, and then go back into braces. This prospect may seem upsetting at first, but when the patient is shown the x-rays with his or her jaws out of alignment and the connection is made to the dozens of symptoms of the TMD that they have, they are grateful to have help.

THE TMJ UNDER STRESS

So, how did the jaws get out of alignment in the first place? It's important to understand that when a person bites down to chew his or her food, the TMJ and surrounding muscles always seek a position to accommodate the best fit of the teeth. The rule is this: Teeth dominate, muscles and joints accommodate, so it stands to reason that the jaw joint will accommodate as well as it can. If the jaw joints and teeth work together in harmony, then the actions of the jaws will operate smoothly and without incident for years, even a lifetime.

Conversely, when the act of chewing forces the jaws out of a healthy position, repeated stress occurs within the joint and the surrounding muscles and nerves. The typical scenario is this: Every time a person bites down in an unhealthy position, the top end of the lower jaw, called the condyle, is forced back too far and pushes into a ligament (called the posterior ligament) that contains nerves and blood vessels. These nerves and blood vessels are constantly under assault and go to areas like the ears, eyes, and even the brain—areas that are vitally important to a person's overall health and happiness. The following anatomical illustration shows the pinching of the nerves and blood vessels that have to pass through the area in the posterior of the jaw joint. There literally is no other area for them to pass through that wouldn't be very vulnerable to other outside pressures or injuries. Unfortunately, they are subject to damage internally from improper condyle placement.

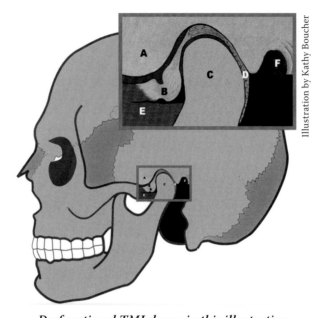

Dysfunctional TMJ shown in this illustration

A=Temporal Bone; B=Disk (showing degeneration); C=Condyle;
D=Posterior Ligament (showing pinched nerves and blood vessels);
E=Lateral Pterygoid Muscle in Spasm; F=Ear Canal

No wonder the symptoms of TMD are so widespread. Similar to having a pinched nerve in your neck, the nerves and blood vessels affected can be painful. Topping the list of the most common problems are headaches, facial pain, problems with the eyes and ears, and even neck problems (for a list of symptoms to track when being treated for TMD, please see the Symptoms Rating Sheet in Appendix B). More recent discoveries point to the fact that even many neurological disorders, such as Parkinson's disease and Tourette's syndrome, can have a direct relationship with TMJ dysfunction. I have included an article, also in Appendix B, for further information on this.

In addition to the compression of the nerves and blood vessels, there is a disc of cartilage within the joint that takes a great deal of abuse as the dysfunction continues. When the lower jaw opens and closes, a clicking or popping sound occurs when the condyle goes on and off the disc. This is by far the most classic sign of TMD. *Clicking jaws are not normal!* As the condyle migrates back and the disc migrates forward, the condyle can get stuck behind the disc, limiting the person's ability to open his or her mouth widely. The clicking stops at this point because the condyle is stuck behind the disc. This condition is known as a "closed-lock" and can make eating anything a real pain. Over time, if left untreated, this disc of cartilage gets stretched further away from its normal position and becomes worn and deformed. Even though the disc's condition has deteriorated, the clicking and popping sounds may diminish over time as the disc gets smaller and smaller and more and more deformed. In more advanced stages, grating sounds (called crepitis) occur when the condyle finally wears through the ligament and results in bone-on-bone contact when a person opens and closes his or her mouth. Over time, this progressive deterioration of the TMJ makes the condition more debilitative and more difficult to treat.

NASAL OBSTRUCTION
CAN EXACERBATE TMJ DYSFUNCTION

A far less obvious, but important, source of stress on the jaw joints is any type of nasal obstruction that results in a mouth-breathing habit, the causes and effects of which are discussed in detail in Chapter 6. The muscles that open the jaw for mouth breathing pull the lower jaw back at the same time, putting further pressure on the TMJs and causing them to go out of alignment. This is why mouth breathing is a contributing factor to TMD.

FORWARD HEAD POSTURE

Another reflex action occurs with the retruded lower jaw: the head moves forward as the body attempts to compensate for the position of the lower jaw. Forward head posture is a condition well known by chiropractors and physical therapists and will be discussed in more detail in Chapter 8. What these well-meaning practitioners sometimes don't realize, however, is that the forward head posture they work so hard to correct cannot be successfully corrected unless the reflex action of an overbite or mouth-breathing habits are eliminated. I personally have never seen a mouth-breather patient who didn't have a forward head posture—and I have been looking closely for the last twenty-six years. Healthcare professionals working in the head and neck area need to work together for the patient's benefit. Poor head posture, which begins with straining of the neck muscles and leads to the loss of the normal curvature of the neck, can lead to a host of painful neck and back problems, oftentimes leading to a stooped posture in old age.

So, contrary to popular belief, TMJ disorders can affect youngsters, the major cause being that which you have seen referred to as the trapped lower jaw. If not detected and corrected, this condition can become worse over time, resulting in a serious TMJ problem in adulthood. It is estimated that as many as eighty million Americans suffer from TMD at some point in their lives. The case of Michelle, told in Chapter 2, is a story heard all too commonly from the adult patients seeking help for their TMJ problems.

The following is the story of a young lady, Dee, who I was introduced to in an unusual way. I had a chance meeting with her mother at a church gathering. She seemed to take a profound interest in what I did for a living as our discussion progressed from routine orthodontics to my emphasis on correcting TMJ dysfunctions. She told me her daughter was going through orthodontics and that her orthodontist felt she was about ready to get her braces off. However, Dee was having a lot of pain in her jaws and they were constantly clicking. She told me that her orthodontist didn't seem to think this was a problem and thought that things would probably settle down once the braces were off. "Does this sound okay to you, Dr. Lauson?" she asked anxiously. When I answered, "Definitely not, this is a problem that needs to be dealt with before orthodontics is completed," she asked me to evaluate her daughter.

My evaluation of Dee, fourteen years old as a new patient, revealed several things of note. Interestingly, her teeth appeared very well aligned and I could see that the orthodontics was performed to a high standard. The teeth appeared ready for brace removal. However, investigation of the x-rays taken revealed that Dee's jaw joints were significantly out of alignment. She had substantial tenderness in many of the muscles that controlled movements of her jaw, as well as in her jaw joints themselves. Both dental arches were moderately constricted. Of the many symptoms I assessed, the major ones included headaches, jaw and jaw-joint pain, clicking, popping, and locking of the jaw joints, difficulty opening the jaws, dizziness, loss of concentration, visual disturbances, and clenching of the teeth. The fact that Dee's braces were about to be removed, and she had substantial pain and dysfunction in her jaw joints, meant that she was being set up for a life of pain with no help in sight.

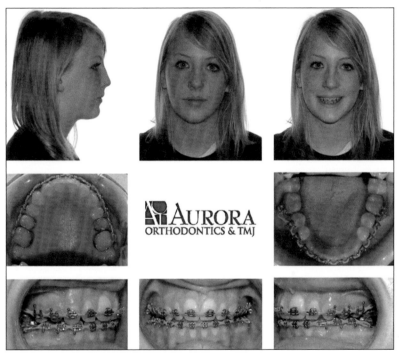

Pretreatment photos

Because treatment to correct Dee's jaw joints would take several months before I could even address the correction of her narrow arches, which would take several additional months, we decided to remove Dee's braces and replace them later. The treatment of her jaw-joint dysfunction was very successful and her associated symptom levels were reduced by over 90% within four months. Her jaw joints were now operating normally with no clicking, popping, locking, or pain.

Once her symptoms levels were down and the TMJs were functioning properly, we began to address the orthodontic and orthopedic concerns. You can see in the photos that after the TMJ correction her upper jaw was considerably narrower than her lower teeth, and, of course, nothing else matched either. First, we needed to widen her upper jaw and did so using FFO. This took about four months, and then we were able to put braces back. They were used to finish correcting the position of the teeth to match the new, more ideal position of the jaw joints. Treatment with the braces was completed within sixteen months.

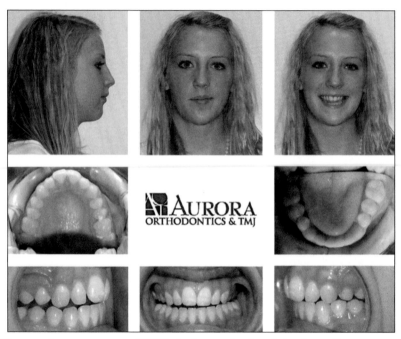

Photos after treatment of TMD, before orthodontic/orthopedic treatment

It is easy to follow the sequence of events here and understand that the previous orthodontist was at a loss as to how to correct this child's TMJ problem. Had I not chanced to meet Dee's mother, the problem would not have been addressed, potentially causing many additional years of pain and discomfort.

It is very important that those doing orthodontic treatment become well versed in the treatment of TMJ dysfunctions because these disorders commonly arise as the bite changes during orthodontic treatment. This knowledge allows the dental professional to responsibly correct this very common problem in the patients he or she treats.

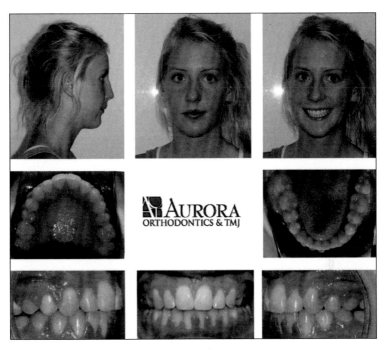

Photos taken at the time of brace removal

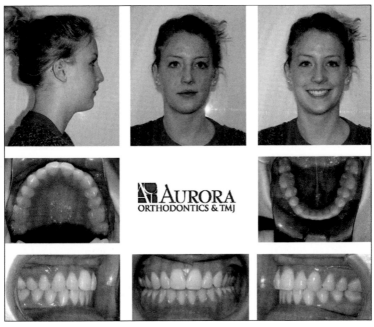

Eighteen months after brace removal

While home from college, Dee recently came back to our office and shared the following thoughts:

Before I started seventh grade in 2004, I got my braces on. I remember being so excited to have braces and to have my teeth fixed. Toward the end of eighth grade, a year and a half later, I started noticing that my jaw would lock. There was one time where I wasn't able to open my mouth fully for almost a week and a half and it was very painful. The times that my jaw was not locked, it would click, get stuck, and I wasn't able to chew without pain. During this time, my former orthodontist had me wearing rubber bands to fix my overbite. I told him numerous times of the painful locking and clicking in my jaw, but he said it was normal and it wasn't a problem and it would go away and I just had to deal with it. I was also experiencing extremely bad headaches almost daily. After a few months of dealing with this, my mom got concerned and tried to talk to the orthodontist and he told her the same thing, I just had to deal with it.

At this time, my mom talked with her friend, Dr. Lauson. He said that this is NOT okay and he suggested that we come to his office for consultation. After talking with Dr. Lauson, and him reviewing the x-rays and a questionnaire that I filled out, I was diagnosed with TMJ. He explained what all of this meant, why I was in such pain, and suggested a new treatment plan. I became a patient of Dr. Lauson that day.

Dr. Lauson removed my braces and said that he was going to work on the problem at hand, the TMJ. He would concentrate on straightening my teeth later. I was fitted with and wore an orthotic and given muscle relaxing treatments every two weeks for a little less than a year. I started noticing a difference right away. My jaw wasn't locking as much and my headaches were subsiding. After a while, I got my braces back on and my teeth began to move into their proper positions. In the spring of 2009, my senior year in high school, I got my braces off and I can remember how excited I was. After five years I was so glad to get them off, and also be completely pain free. I am so grateful for Dr. Lauson. He really listened to what I was saying, was very concerned at my pain level, and explained everything he was doing and why. He is always very kind, is interested in what I am up to. I am extremely grateful that he was there for me.

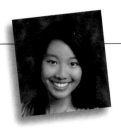

CHAPTER 8

Key #5: Ideal Head Posture

Now let's explore the influence of teeth on head posture. As it turns out, teeth have a lot of influence, bad and good, on a person's head posture. Fortunately, with early intervention, many of the problems associated with poor posture can be avoided simply by addressing the displacement of the lower jaw and teeth.

As we know, when the jaw is retruded, the head moves into a forward head posture in an attempt to remain in balance, consequently putting a great deal of strain on the muscles of the neck and upper back. In the medical community, it is believed that every inch the head is carried forward from an ideal posture is the equivalent of adding ten pounds to the neck's muscle load. This has an effect on the vertebrae in the neck, ultimately leading to the loss of cervical lordosis (the normal curvature of the neck). This unhealthy condition—sometimes referred to as a "straight neck" or "military neck"—results in a loss of mobility of the neck. If one can't look over his shoulder at the car behind him, chances are he has lost some of the curvature and mobility of his neck.

Chronic forward head posture has also been shown not only to reduce a person's quality of life by causing many related ailments, but also even to reduce a person's life expectancy. It affects wide-ranging physiological functions, from breathing to hormonal production. Due to tension on the spinal cord, its coverings, and associated blood vessels, abnormal spinal curvatures can also lead to spinal dislocations and degenerative neurological conditions over time.

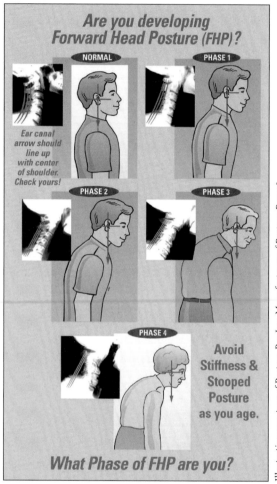

This illustration shows the progression of forward head posture and the loss of curvature (even reverse curvature, called kyphosis) of the neck spine.

How is this possible? Because of the nervous system's influence on the body, spinal misalignments and malfunctions can lead to or aggravate many seemingly unrelated but common conditions not typically associated with the spine. The slumping indicative of a forward head or body posture has been found to be directly related to current or potential spinal dysfunction, pain, and general ill health—a true sign of old age (skeletal age, that is!). Researchers continually study and confirm the far-reaching effects of abnormal spinal function on the areas of immune response, aging, hormonal production, and even genetics.

Although this fact is virtually unknown and ignored in medical literature, early treatment of dental malocclusions, such as overbites and constricted upper jaws, can have a very positive influence on a person's overall postural development. As stated earlier, if problems such as an overbite or mouth-breathing habit are not corrected (and in conjunction with proposed physical therapy or chiropractic treatment), the poor head posture will not be successfully treated. This is certainly one area of health that a person with knowledge can use to actively, positively, and profoundly impact his or her overall body health. The importance of early orthodontic intervention as recommended in The Lauson System, if indicated, can have a very positive effect to help assure proper postural development.

The following young lady's treatment shows how this very important key comes into play in her orthodontic treatment. Jamie was eight years old when she came to my office for a routine orthodontic evaluation. She had upper and lower jaw constrictions and was developing crowding in both dental arches. I could see that the crowding in her lower front teeth was soon to get worse, as the last remaining lower incisor was due to come in and there was no room for it. Her lower jaw was slightly recessed (Class II molar relationship) and there was clicking in her right TMJ. She had a loss of the natural curvature of her neck (see Chapter 8) and a forward head posture.

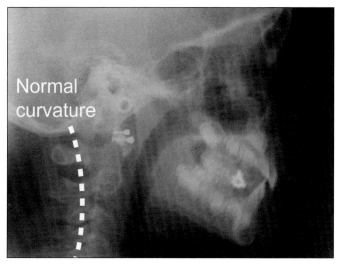

X-ray showing the loss of curvature in Jamie's neck

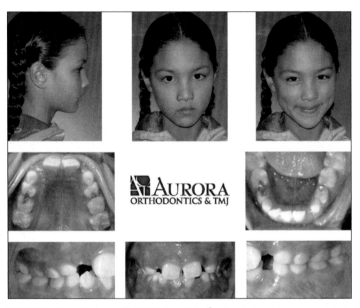

Pretreatment photos

When I initially began treating Jamie, I used a removable expansion appliance. Unfortunately, the fit of the appliance was not as precise as I would have liked and patient cooperation was not great. After several months, we stopped treatment until more of the permanent teeth came in. A number of months later, she presented with a large cavity on the upper-right primary second molar. We referred her to her family dentist to have the tooth removed as we were going to use a treatment appliance that would hold the space.

Because we had not completed the entire upper arch development during the previous phase I treatment, we elected to use an upper 3-way sagittal appliance (see Appendix A for description of all treatment appliances), so we could gain the room necessary for the upper cuspid teeth that were blocked out. While this was happening, new bone was forming, which allowed the upper front teeth to come forward. This in turn had the additional positive effects of allowing her lower jaw to come more forward, helping to correct her head posture. With very good patient cooperation this time, seven months later we placed a full set of braces. Ten months after the braces were placed, we completed our treatment. Jamie's TMD issue and forward head posture were resolved and her jaw came forward into a more natural and ideal position.

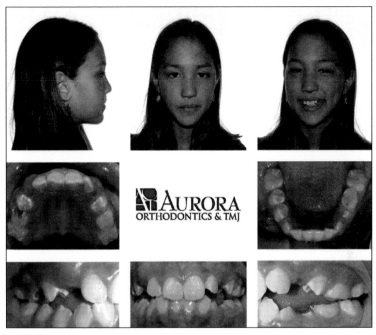

Progress photos before phase II orthodontic treatment

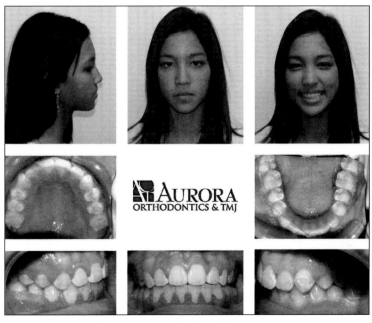

Photos at completion of treatment

Upon seeing Jamie three years after her treatment, the corrections made have remained stable.

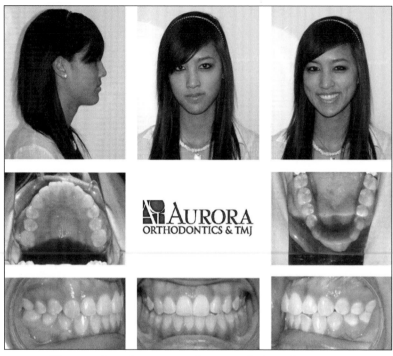

Photos taken three years after completion of treatment

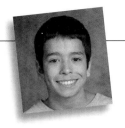

CHAPTER 9

Key #6: Avoidance of Obstructive Sleep Apnea

Obstructive sleep apnea is another one of those conditions that doesn't seem obvious for inclusion in a book about children's orthodontics. As you have already seen with the keys for Healthy TMJ Function and Ideal Head Posture, addressing problems within the mouth has a farther-reaching impact than simply what the teeth look like and their function. Obstructive sleep apnea is another condition that can be affected by orthodontic treatment for better or worse.

Let's start by describing just what obstructive sleep apnea (OSA) is. OSA is the most common type of sleep disorder (among several types) and occurs when a person goes to sleep lying on his or her back and the back of the tongue rests too far back in the throat area. This can cause an obstruction of the air passageway, resulting in the stopping of airflow during breathing.

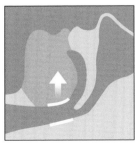
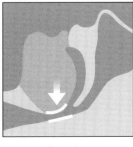
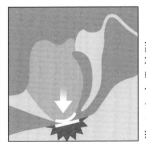

Normal   *Snoring*   *OSA*

Illustration by Todd Gilmore

This restriction results in a lack of oxygen being delivered to the brain and usually causes the person to either wake up briefly or shift so that the blockage is relieved and air can again flow. It is called an apnea event if the stoppage lasts ten seconds or longer. Repeated events like this throughout the night are defined as obstructive sleep apnea and are classified as mild, moderate, or severe, depending on the age of the patient and the number of apnea events that occur per hour of sleep. It is considered very serious if a child has even a small number of apnea events because of their immediate effects and because this progressive disorder intensifies with age.

It has been well established that OSA creates cardiovascular stress, which leads to strokes or heart attacks (with the possibility of death). OSA is also associated with many seemingly unrelated degenerative diseases, including pulmonary and systemic hypertension, diabetes, kidney disease, and ADD/ADHD. Studies show that a person with OSA has an average of twelve years cut off his or her life expectancy. It is known that as many as seventy-five million people in North America suffer from OSA; because of its widespread prevalence, it is a major health problem.

In recent years, the lack of restful sleep and the resultant daytime drowsiness have been well documented. Now more motor vehicle accident deaths result from drowsiness than from drunk drivers. One hundred thousand deadly truck accidents occur each year because of a truck driver falling asleep at the wheel, and each time a crash occurs it takes two to four other people with it. In the news are stories of an epidemic of serious accidents caused by this daytime drowsiness, not the least of which includes a major problem with our air-traffic controllers falling asleep on the job. Investigations of some of the most famous human-error accidents, including Exxon Valdez, Chernobyl, Three Mile Island, and the Challenger disaster, have all been linked to drowsiness on the job due to lack of appropriate sleep. But as you will see, this does not have to be the problem that it is, as the prevention, and even reversal, of OSA can be accomplished with the techniques discussed here and used in The Lauson System.

OSA typically starts early in life as a mild obstruction and generally is accompanied by snoring. As the years pass by, if left unattended, the obstruction can progress into a sleep apnea problem. Although OSA is typically thought of as a problem for middle-aged, overweight males, the truth is that OSA can and does exist in a very broad range of the population. Young and old, male and female, large and small all have the possibility of OSA. When a person has OSA, which is confirmed by an overnight sleep study at a sleep center facility with a sleep physician, the primary recommendation for a person with OSA is to use a continuous positive air pressure (CPAP) machine. This device literally pushes air through a person's nose all night long to give him or her much needed oxygen as he or she sleeps. A secondary device, especially for those who are CPAP-intolerant, is an oral (dental) airway appliance used while sleeping. This device works by holding the jaw forward, which creates more room behind the tongue for air to flow.

During childhood, OSA can exist because of enlarged tonsils, adenoids, or any other obstruction that results in mouth breathing. OSA has been linked as a cause of ADHD and even SIDS. When this airway obstruction is discovered, it must be removed right away, regardless of the age of the patient. A child with a deep overbite and a retruded, or recessed, lower jaw has a big, developing problem that needs correction. A child with any nasal obstruction must have it eliminated.

A young person with a narrow upper jaw and developing overbite is already set up for future OSA. If the narrow upper jaw and overbite are not corrected in the ideal manner—by enlarging the constricted upper jaw and freeing up the lower jaw to come forward into the ideal position—the die is cast for OSA. An enlightened orthodontist or dentist performing orthodontics should recognize this fact and be instrumental in the prevention of a future OSA condition. This is a huge opportunity for proper progressive orthodontic treatment to eliminate the future problem of OSA and to give a lifelong benefit to the patient.

A nagging flaw in traditional orthodontic education exists. As a result of the removal of permanent teeth, the jaws are left in their less-than-ideal narrow state and a restriction of the upper-air passageway that exists is made worse by diminishing the airflow through it. This happens to be the first choke point in the airflow system of the head and neck. The removal of teeth also causes the lower jaw to remain trapped in a retruded position, causing the airflow to the throat area (the second and final choke point) to also be lessened. Consequently, the removal of permanent teeth has a twofold effect, making a future of OSA much more likely.

The Lauson System of orthodontic treatment used in young patients to prevent the development of OSA (and TMJ and neck problems as well) is as follows:

1. Widen the upper jaw to an ideal full arch form (Key #1)
2. Make sure any nasal passageway obstruction is cleared (Key #2)
3. Encourage the lower jaw to grow forward to balance with the upper jaw (Key #3)

The goal of this treatment is to prevent the problem of OSA from developing later in life. Hopefully you see a pattern developing here: that all of the keys to The Lauson System are compatible, synergistic, and complementary; they build on each other. When one key is achieved, it is easier to achieve others. If any of the keys are ignored, then the patient suffers in one way or another. Yes, many people live their whole lives without having the advantage of what this treatment has to offer; however, when people in the future seek help from an enlightened orthodontist or dentist performing orthodontics, they may be offered the full benefit of the nine keys.

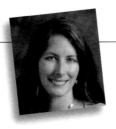

CHAPTER 10

Key #7: Ideal Lower Facial Symmetry

Just what then is symmetry? A definition from Encarta Dictionary is as follows:

> *sym.me.try* 1. The property of being the same or corresponding on both sides of a central dividing line 2. Harmony or beauty of form that results from balanced proportions

Basically, symmetry means one side of an object is the mirror image of the opposite side, resulting in harmony and beauty. Therefore, it is important to understand that everything talked about here is consistent for creating the most symmetrical result to the greatest extent possible. It is also important to understand that complete facial symmetry is not realistic; virtually no face is completely symmetrical. Even the recognized movie star Jennifer Lopez, although a great example of facial symmetry, still shows a slight asymmetry. The picture on the left is her actual portrait. The other two pictures show the mirror images of the left and the right halves of her face, respectively.

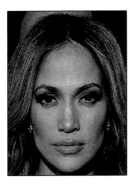 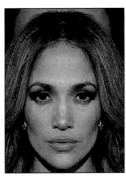 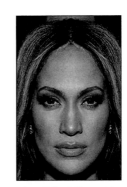

Actual Photo   ***Left-Side Mirror Image***   ***Right-Side Mirror Image***

It has long been a goal of orthodontics, as well as maxillofacial surgery, to create facial symmetry. Therefore, it is also one of the nine keys to lower facial harmony as presented in The Lauson System.

HISTORY OF FACIAL SYMMETRY

Charles Feng, of Stanford University, discussed the history of facial symmetry by using the example of Helen of Troy (instigator of the Trojan War), who was known for her incredible beauty. She was not celebrated for her kindness or her intellect, but for her physical perfection. Regarding facial beauty, Plato wrote of "golden proportions," stating (among other dimensions for importance) the width of an ideal face should be two-thirds its length, while a nose should be no longer than the distance between the eyes. Plato's golden proportions, however, haven't quite held up to the rigors of modern psychological and biological research—though there is credence in the ancient Greeks' attempts to determine a fundamental symmetry that humans find attractive. Today, it has been scientifically proven that symmetry is inherently attractive to the human eye.

In these modern times, applying the stringent conditions of today's scientific methods, researchers believe symmetry shows that the ancient Greeks were on the right track.

"Facial symmetry is one of a number of traits associated with health, physical attractiveness and beauty of a person."

—Science Daily

Over the years, many studies have verified that facial symmetry is dominant in our perception of beauty. In a segment entitled "Five Elements of Attractiveness" from the Oprah Winfrey Show on August 14, 2009, it was stated that "physical attraction may be as old as time, but new studies are beginning to uncover the science behind sex appeal. Unexpected factors—like smell, *facial symmetry* [emphasis mine], voice pitch, financial stability and kissing prowess—just might have more to do with your choice of mate than anyone ever expected." Studies have gone so far as to compare identical twins from a beauty standpoint: the more symmetric the face, the more beautiful each was rated.

STANDARDS FOR COSMETIC SURGERY –
IDEAL FACIAL DIMENSIONS

The following is another report of interest, which explores techniques that many plastic surgeons use to determine ideal facial proportions. Beauty is not an exact science; nonetheless, according to some plastic surgeons there is a specific proportion system where the ideal face tends to hover. This system includes facial height, width, and symmetry. The face is evaluated from its frontal view and then its profile view to evaluate symmetrical proportions. Other assessments are made for contours such as the cheekbones, chin, and nose.

The standards commonly used to measure facial symmetry are shown in the following illustrations. The face is divided into thirds, as shown. In order to have the best facial balance, each third should be as equal as possible. If any section of the face is out of proportion in relation to the others, the result is less pleasing to the eye.

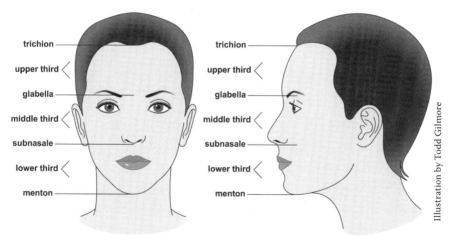

Horizontal Facial Thirds – Front   *Horizontal Facial Thirds – Profile*

Another method to measure symmetry is to divide the face into fifths, using the width of the eye from corner to corner as a point of measurement.

From the very outside edge of one ear to the other, the face ideally is five eye widths apart. The width of the base of the nose, at the nostrils (or ala), ideally is one-fifth of the face, or one eye width.

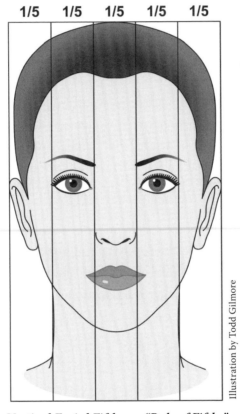

1/5   1/5   1/5   1/5   1/5

Illustration by Todd Gilmore

Vertical Facial Fifths, or "Rule of Fifths"

A study done in 2007 by a team of researchers at California State University at Northridge specifically reveals the importance of lower jaw symmetry. It suggests that lower jaw symmetry is the most important aspect of facial symmetry. The study results show that "increased symmetry of the jaw line increases perceived levels of facial attractiveness, whereas other areas of facial symmetry were not rated as high in importance."[1]

---

[1] Maria Chan, Natalie Johnson, Ayelet Linden, and Argineh Margharian, "The Relationship Between Various Measurements of Facial Symmetry and Ratings of Physical Attractiveness." (California State University, Northridge) May 17, 2007, http://www.csun.edu

FACIAL ASYMMETRY,
A TRICKY PROBLEM

Facial asymmetries are among the most challenging problems for an orthodontist to resolve. When a lower-facial asymmetry is observed in a patient, it is commonly thought that it is a result of unequal growth in the right and left halves of the face. This is particularly true of asymmetries in the lower jaw.

Let's look back to the origin of the problem, and ask the question, "What circumstances were present in the first place?" During the formative years, a common problem that occurs is that the lower jaw shifts off to one side or the other due to what is called a unilateral-posterior crossbite. A crossbite is defined as the upper teeth hitting on the inside of the lower teeth. When a crossbite doesn't allow the back teeth to comfortably come together in order to chew, a person accommodates by habitually shifting his or her jaw to the right or left every time he or she bites down. The displacement of the jaw to one side results in lower facial asymmetry, as shown in the following illustrations.

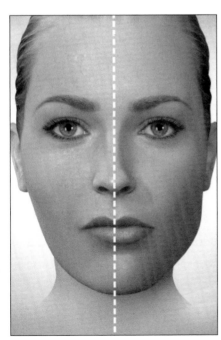 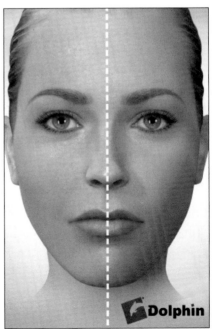

Illustration courtesy Dolphin® Imaging & Management Solutions

Lower-Jaw Asymmetry to the Right *Lower Jaw Centered*

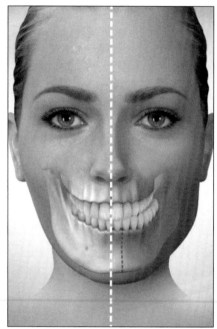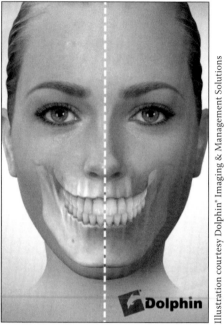

Illustration courtesy Dolphin® Imaging & Management Solutions

Note the midline marked by the blue dotted line on the left
illustration showing the asymmetry of the lower jaw to the right

An accepted explanation in traditional orthodontics for this asymmetry is that the lower jaw has grown less on the side in the direction where the jaw has shifted. This may be true in some cases, but not true in others. Something very subtle can be going on here as well. Because the TMJ is highly flexible, it allows the lower jaw to shift back too much on one or both sides as it grows. This is the most common reason for TMD and explains why the pain in the jaw joint may be experienced on one side but not necessarily on the other. So, when the lower jaw has shifted to one side, it can be perceived as a lower-jaw asymmetry, when it is actually a displacement of the entire lower jaw.

This condition has fooled many orthodontists and oral surgeons alike, as the traditional approach to solving these problems has been primarily surgical in nature. Some surgeries have been performed to correct the asymmetrical growth, while the real problem has been the shifting of the jaw to the side. The surgical correction lengthens the lower jaw on the seemingly deficient side and, unfortunately, can leave that side with the jaw joint out of alignment causing TMD. X-rays of the jaw joints must be taken to see the whole picture before surgery is performed. This helps to determine the proper alignment of the TMJs and helps to answer the burning question as to whether surgery is warranted. In many cases the lower-jaw asymmetry may be addressed by first correcting the TMJ alignment so that any remaining mandibular asymmetry is manageable without surgery. In other cases where a true skeletal asymmetry has developed, surgery may be the only viable option. The key here is to attempt to correct the problem as early as possible since delaying corrective treatment may take away the nonsurgical option. Other facial asymmetries, such as in the midface, may be helped with creative FFO treatment, but for many facial asymmetries, surgery may still be the best answer.

The following case illustrates how asymmetrical development of the lower face can occur. Emily was seven and a half years old when she arrived at our office as a new patient. Her upper jaw had a severe constriction, causing substantial crowding of the teeth. Because her lower jaw was only mildly constricted, the mismatch of her upper and lower teeth caused her lower jaw to shift to her left when she bit down, as you can see in the photos below.

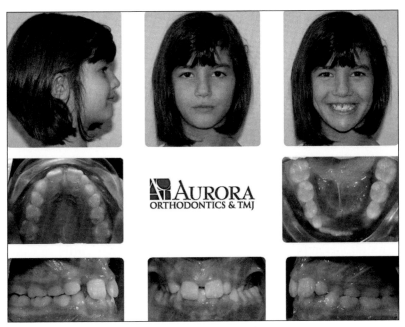

Pretreatment photos

Although her jaw joints checked out normally, due to the unevenness of the bite, there were sensitive areas in the muscles that allowed her to chew as they were having to work extra hard to do their job. An expander called a quad helix (see Appendix A for description of all treatment appliances) was used to gain the necessary expansion on the upper jaw. The expander worked its wonders and the expansion was completed within the first six months. We then waited for another six months until the upper and lower front four teeth had come into her mouth. Braces were then placed to complete the alignment of the front teeth over the next four months, for a total of fifteen months of treatment.

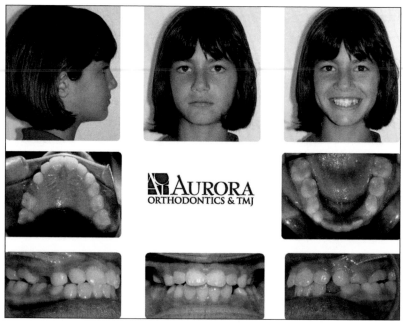

Photos after completion of phase I treatment

The treatment performed as an initial phase treatment reached the objective of correcting a deficiency in the upper jaw in order to establish a much better symmetry, as shown in the photos taken at the end of this first phase of treatment. Although this initial phase of treatment did not completely correct the asymmetry, in the future at around age eleven or twelve, the final phase of treatment will ultimately address any remaining concerns with symmetry and her bite. The corrections made also eliminated the need for removal of any permanent teeth and minimized treatment challenges in the future.

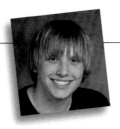

CHAPTER 11

Key #8: Elimination of Adverse Oral Habits

It is well known in the dental field that adverse oral habits, such as thumb sucking, can have a very negative effect on the facial development of a growing child. This is due to adverse pressures exerted during the execution of the habit. The longer the pressure exists each day and the more strength that is exerted in the affected area, the more profound the negative result is. These habits, allowed to continue uncontrolled over a number of years, have far-reaching effects. Each of these habits must be eliminated. The following is a good list of habits to avoid:

1. MOUTH BREATHING:

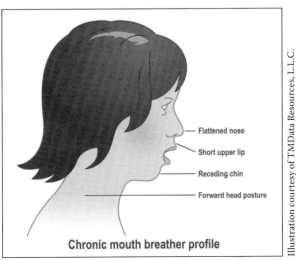

— Flattened nose

— Short upper lip

— Receding chin

— Forward head posture

Chronic mouth breather profile

Illustration courtesy of TMData Resources, L.L.C.

Chapter 5 discussed how destructive an obstructed nasal passageway can be, forcing a person to breathe through his or her mouth, and how this habit can be eliminated. Consequently, I will not go into detail here.

2. IMPROPER TONGUE PLACEMENT:

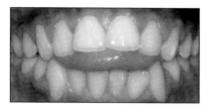 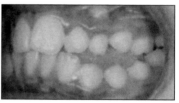

Anterior Tongue Thrust   *Lateral or Side Tongue Thrust*

Adverse swallowing habits or poor posturing of the tongue can have a profound effect on the stability of the teeth and, if left unchecked, can really ruin a beautiful orthodontic result. How does this happen? This is an example of the chicken and egg debate, where the dentist wonders whether the open bites shown are the cause or the result of adverse tongue posture. It has been my experience that poor tongue-posture habits are the result of any number of factors, including a mouth-breathing problem, too-narrow of an upper dental arch form, a larger-than-ideal tongue size, or a combination of these factors. Sometimes the habit is a residual one that persists after proper treatment. This causes an open bite to develop, as the orthodontic result is not completely stable in the months immediately after brace removal.

3. BOTTLE-FEEDING:

While not considered a bad habit by most, bottle-feeding a baby instead of breast-feeding is another way to develop an adverse tongue habit. The suckling instinct is as natural as eating—for a baby, of course, that's just what it is. The suckling instinct is also a powerful exercise of jaws and joints. The problem is that the suckling instinct can take many detours, which impact mouth and health. In various studies, bottle-feeding has been associated with causing forward-thrusts of the tongue that, over time, lead to irregularities of the teeth and bite. Why is that? It's because of the way babies relate to the placement of the bottle into the mouth and to the artificial nipple. To make for easier feeding (and satisfied consumers), manufacturers oftentimes give the nipple an unnaturally strong flow. Here's an example of the law of unintended consequences kicking in: once the baby is satisfied, she tries to push away the artificial nipple—still gushing milk—with her tongue. This sequence, happening multiple times a day from the first day of a child's life, can lay the groundwork for a tongue-thrusting habit, which in turn negatively impacts the formation of the jaws and teeth.

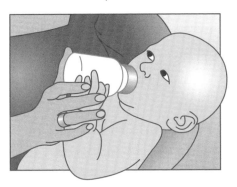

4. THUMB AND FINGER SUCKING:

Thumb- and finger-sucking habits can also include lip sucking, which over a period of time can cause the bone structure of the upper and lower jaw to change significantly. It's a fundamental human activity, one that can even begin in the womb.

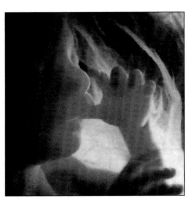

Ultrasound technology has shown that many developing babies have a thumb in their mouth.

Of all humanity's behavioral quirks, one of the more common—not to mention controversial—is thumb (or finger) sucking. When a newborn in a crib sucks his thumb, people coo, "Isn't that cute?" but when that cute baby is age six and still sucking his thumb, he's scolded for not being a "big boy."

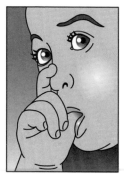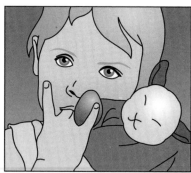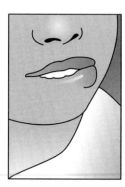

Thumb, Finger, and Lip Sucking Habits

Everyone from psychologists to parents has an opinion on thumb sucking. Some consider it a natural source of comfort; others condemn it as an emotional crutch. Dentists, perhaps more than anyone else, see the devastating effects of prolonged thumb sucking. Therefore, as part of any orthodontic plan, this adverse habit should be addressed. If left unchecked, it will cause instability of any orthodontic treatment and make a good orthodontic result impossible.

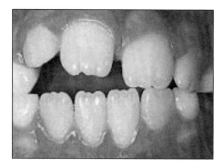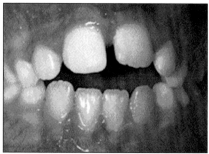

Examples of changes of teeth with
adverse thumb, finger, or tongue habits

5. SWALLOWING TOOTHPASTE:

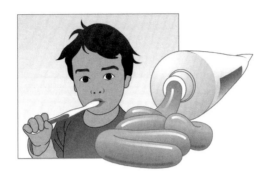

Typically the swallowing of toothpaste is a young child's problem and is a result of a child using too much toothpaste and swallowing once the brushing is finished. Fluoride ingested into a child's body can cause a chronic condition called fluorosis. This discoloration and pitting occurs during development of the teeth before they erupt into the mouth.

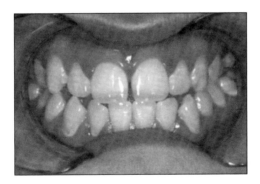

Surface contact of fluoride against the teeth is safe and effective in preventing tooth decay. However, fluoride is considered highly toxic if ingested in anything greater than minute quantities. Toothpaste should be used in tiny amounts and always spit out (never ingested). If the amount of fluoride ingested is extremely high, it can cause fluoride toxicity, which can lead to bone and spinal problems and even death. Like most minerals and compounds, swallowing enough fluoride can kill or severely harm a person. Although rare in the US, this is common in some small villages in countries where water naturally contains large deposits of fluoride.

6. TEETH CLENCHING AND GRINDING:

Teeth clenching and grinding are common problems that are sometimes reduced simply by a making a person aware of the habit.

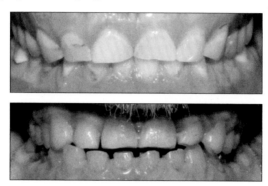

Examples of teeth with excessive wear due to clenching and grinding

Unfortunately, this habit is most likely the result of more serious problems. It can be the result of TMJ dysfunction and a bite that is not ideal, but new evidence shows that it also can be caused from OSA, theorized as being caused by a person habitually moving his or her jaw forward to protect his or her airway. Many times the dentist prescribes a night-guard appliance, worn when sleeping, to protect the teeth from wear. When either TMD or OSA is present, this is a short-term solution; a more permanent solution is accomplished with an orthotic for TMJ correction, followed by maxillary expansion to help OSA, and braces or Invisalign to finish.

7. CHEWING ON FOREIGN OBJECTS:

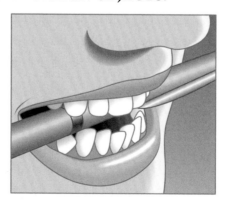

Oral habits, such as chewing on pens, pencils, and even fingernails, have negative effects over time that can cause excessive wear on the surfaces of teeth. These habits can also lead to more serious problems, such as TMJ disorders, because of the continuous stress placed on the jaw joints.

8. GUM CHEWING:

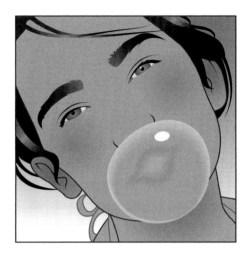

It has been shown that the very common and socially accepted habit of gum chewing (if chewed on a regular, daily basis) can have a substantially negative effect on TMJ function. Excessive chewing of substances other than food (including chewing tobacco products) can also have a negative effect. When treating patients with TMD, these habits must be eliminated.

9. JAW PLAYING:

The seemingly harmless, nervous habit of jutting the jaw around excessively can also have a very harmful effect on the TMJs over time. This may be a transitory habit a child picks up, but eventually gives up.

10. RESTING CHIN ON PALM:

A person's habit of leaning his or her chin on the palm of his or her hand can have a negative effect on the person's TMJ function over a period of time.

This habit may be related to poor head posture, which pulls on the neck muscles; resting the head to relieve the straining of the neck then places additional strain on the jaw. When a person leans on a supporting object (palm of hand), he or she does so to give some relief of the straining in the neck.

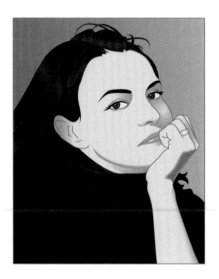

11. ICE CHEWING:

Chewing ice or eating hard objects like jawbreakers (aptly named!) has been linked to a much higher incidence of TMD. This habit can cause significant damage to teeth, including fracturing, which can lead to the need for extensive restorations, such as crowns.

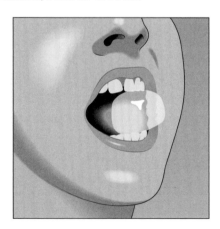

Many of these problems can be successfully addressed when a person simply becomes aware of the problem in the first place and asks for help from a local dental or orthodontic office. Some habits, of course, can be very difficult to break. For a person who has a great deal of difficulty in breaking any of these destructive habits and needs closer one-on-one supervision, a dentist or orthodontist can refer him or her to professionals that work in speech pathology, myofunctional therapy, or orofacial myology. These specialists can be of tremendous help in eliminating these habits.

CASE STUDY SHOWING THE DESTRUCTIVE NATURE OF POOR ORAL HABITS

Patty came to my office as a fourteen-year-old with significant crowding and upper arch constriction. She also had an anterior open bite, which means that she only made contact on her back teeth; the front teeth didn't make contact at all. This created a lot of trauma to the back teeth where she was hitting. Patty had the adverse oral habit of an anterior tongue thrust, which was the primary cause of the open bite. She also had a partial nasal obstruction that caused her to be a mouth breather. She exhibited tightness and tenderness of many neck muscles due to a forward head posture, a result of the mouth-breathing habit. The pretreatment pictures show that a distortion of the bone structure of the upper jaw existed due to the mouth-breathing habit and tongue thrust.

Our treatment took into consideration the adverse habits of mouth breathing and the anterior tongue thrust. We corrected the narrowness of the upper jaw; an upper Schwarz appliance was used for expansion. The appliance included a habit-correction device as a reminder to Patty to keep her tongue properly positioned at the roof of her mouth.

In order to give Patty a more stable final result we referred her to an oral myologist, who worked one-on-one with her in order to completely eliminate the tongue habit. The combined efforts were successful and her treatment was completed in twenty-three months with all nine keys to lower facial harmony achieved. The treatment with FFO eliminated any need for extractions or surgery. The result was a broad, beautiful, and healthy smile.

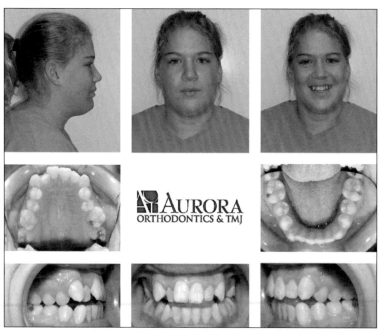

Pretreatment photos showing the anterior open bite and crowding

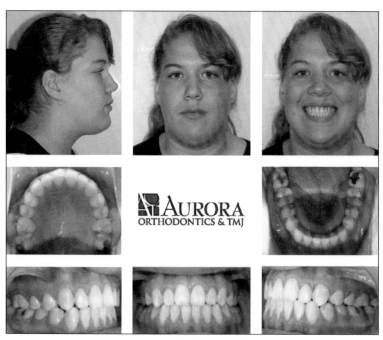

Photos at completion of treatment

Additional comments are as follows: Many orthodontists and oral surgeons consider a skeletal-open-bite case like this—as well as other skeletal problems—as only treatable with a combined orthodontic and surgical approach. However, once FFO principles are understood, surgery can be avoided. Many thousands of skeletal problems like this and other types have been very successfully treated without surgery.

My treatment in this case consisted of two key elements. The first was to correct the orthopedic imbalances present. This required correction of the narrow upper jaw with a functional facial orthopedic expander and then the use of braces.

The second key to success was addressing the adverse tongue and mouth-breathing habits. These habits, once ostensibly broken, could reappear at any time; therefore, recall appointments to assure they hadn't reared their ugly heads were very important. The expansion accomplished during the FFO phase helped to assure the habits would not return because the tongue had adequate space to position itself in the appropriate placement. The combination of the two principles produced a successful and stable result.

---

* Illustrations on pages 91, 92, 93, 94, 95, and 96 done by Todd Gilmore.

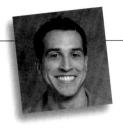

CHAPTER 12

Key #9: Optimal Teeth Positioning

W hat exactly does optimal teeth positioning mean? Since a picture is worth a thousand words, the following illustration shows what we are really talking about.

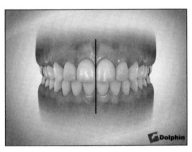 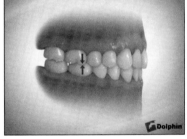

Illustrations courtesy Dolphin®
Imaging & Management Solutions

Midlines together　　　*Proper Class I molar relationship*

So, why is optimal teeth positioning really important? One important aspect is appearance—straight teeth just look more attractive. According to the American Academy of Cosmetic Dentistry, 74% of adults feel that an unattractive smile can hurt a person's chances for career success. In fact, 96% of adults believe an attractive smile makes a person more appealing to members of the opposite sex, and 99.7% believe that a smile is an important social asset. People are rarely born with perfect smiles, but today's technology places great smiles within everyone's reach.

It should go without saying that a great smile is universally accepted as a huge asset to a person in the whole gamut of human endeavors, from business to romance. It is also established that well-fitting teeth are necessary for a healthy bite and jaw joints. This key of optimal teeth positioning really should be the most predictable goal for orthodontic treatment in that virtually all orthodontists and dentists doing orthodontics have this as their primary goal. There is no conflict here: All orthodontics is performed to straighten teeth.

To put the mission of the orthodontist into historical context, the application of braces has been the primary method of straightening teeth in the United States for over a century. However, in Europe and around the rest of the world, other methods have been used (but even in Europe braces are now commonly used to straighten teeth). In modern orthodontics, braces are individually attached to each tooth with a bonding agent or adhesive. Think of braces as little handles attached to each tooth to control its individual movement. The orthodontist applies gentle pressure to a tooth through the brace in order to move it.

Over a number of months, significant tooth movement takes place to bring the tooth into proper alignment. Various items like wires and rubber bands are used to create the forces to move the teeth. Decades ago, bands around the whole tooth were needed to hold the braces in place, but in recent years orthodontics is done almost entirely with what we call direct-bonded brackets, or braces bonded directly to the teeth. They are advantageous in that they are much easier to clean around, as shown in the photo below.

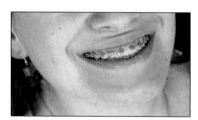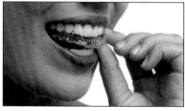

Patients with metal braces and Invisalign® aligners

Significant improvements in treatment have occurred over time. In recent years, many teeth have been straightened with the use of clear, plastic treatment appliances called Invisalign. The Invisalign system consists of a person wearing a series of virtually invisible aligners that apply pressure to the teeth to create the desired movements. These are custom made for each patient and are switched out about every two weeks. After using FFO to achieve more ideal arch form, I have used Invisalign to finish these treatments with a very pleasing result. However, Invisalign will not work on all cases. A doctor proficient in the use of Invisalign will have to evaluate an individual to make that determination. More recently, aligner-based treatment has expanded to more difficult cases, but a percentage of cases still need the conventional braces.

This final key is where orthodontic treatment shines, and has done so for over a hundred years. Aesthetically, this key is important so that the patient has a beautiful, full smile with straight teeth. Perhaps more importantly, in terms of dental health, his or her bite functions properly without undue stress and is stable for a lifetime of use. Time-tested traditional metal braces—and more recently, the innovative alternatives such as Invisalign—are what make the orthodontic treatment live up to the charge, "I want my teeth straight!" Orthodontics, I am sure, will always be best known for work in creating "straight teeth"; but is it enough to just focus on straightening teeth?

Unfortunately, traditional orthodontics typically doesn't take all of the previous keys listed in this book into consideration when treating patients, with the exception of Keys #7 and #8 and the possible exception of Key #2. Straightening teeth without having the other keys as objectives is doing the patient a disservice; ignoring these principles could pave the way for a life of pain and dysfunction. The orthodontist following the principles of The Lauson System has the capacity to substantially elevate the quality of a person's life in many ways.

Once Keys #1–8 are achieved, Key #9 is far less complicated. In fact, this braces or Invisalign phase consumes much less time and energy for the patient and doctor alike. In many cases this final phase is accomplished in half the time it traditionally takes because achieving each of the previous keys allows a more physiologic positioning of the teeth, so the braces require less tooth movement. This is because the expansion creates spacing between teeth, allowing for rapid alignment of the teeth. The savings in time is significant. By contrast, the extraction of permanent teeth that traditional orthodontics calls for to correct crowding can add as much as nine months to overall treatment time just to close the space created. If surgery were included in the treatment plan, an additional four to six months would be needed to allow for healing.

The following case study, although it is not complex, illustrates the ability of Invisalign to make a good smile into a great one and give a result that demonstrates an ideal bite, satisfying the ninth key to lower facial harmony.

When sixteen-year-old Alicia came to our office, she stated that she just wanted a prettier smile. I felt certain that Invisalign Teen® was the answer for her. Alicia was a pretty girl and wanted an even more beautiful smile. When looking at her before pictures, it could be perceived that she didn't need her teeth straightened. After all, her teeth were relatively straight and her bite in the back was right on with a Class I relationship. However, Alicia's dental arch forms were moderately constricted when compared to ideal, and there was slight misalignment of the front teeth. Other findings at the exam revealed some pain on palpation of both the right and left trapezius muscles, which was an early indication of developing TMJ and head-posture problems.

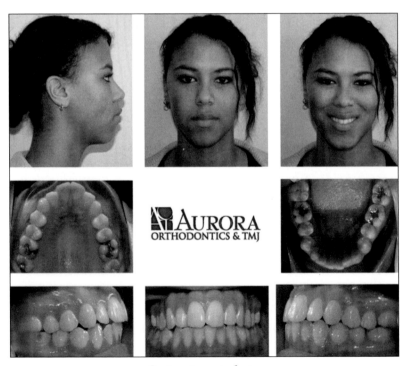

Pretreatment photos

Since her main aesthetic problem was that her narrow arch forms accentuated her front teeth, we gave Alicia the option between widening her smile with upper and lower expansion appliances before her Invisalign Teen treatment or to just going directly into the aligners, where we would be limited in our overall expansion. She elected to do the expanders first, so we started our treatment with FFO expansion, which took about four months before going to the aligners. The result of the expansion is shown in the following pictures.

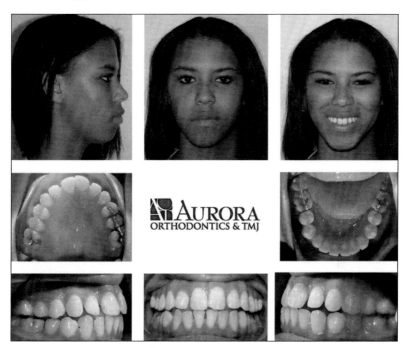

Postexpansion photos, overcorrection leaving spaces,
prior to closing with Invisalign Teen®

Once we were well into the aligners, it became apparent that the use of the aligners had freed up the lower jaw to come slightly forward, causing her teeth to hit first in the front. This is typical in cases where the TMJs have gotten out of position and head posture is forward of normal. We corrected the teeth with a combination of the aligners, and she wore rubber bands so that as the Invisalign correction was taking place, better alignment of the jaw joints was also taking place. After looking at the final pictures shown next, it is evident that an enhancement was accomplished and the result was terrific. Alicia's result qualifies as ideal, which exemplifies the ninth and final key to lower facial harmony.

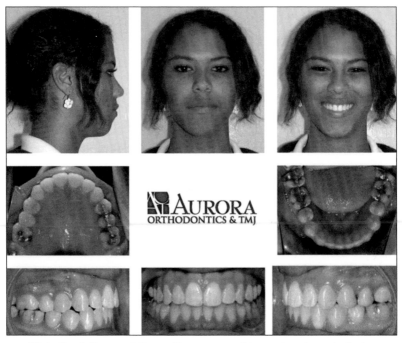

Note the fullness of the smile compared to pretreatment photos

In summary, it is safe to say that orthodontists believe that there is more to a good bite than just the beauty of the smile. When performing any orthodontic correction, the ultimate objective of The Lauson System is to create a beautiful, full smile with proper facial balance, along with a bite that functions properly and is stable over a lifetime. All the other keys, in conjunction with Key #9, allow the dentist or orthodontist to achieve all the previously stated goals of beauty and harmony. The case studies in Part III continue to graphically illustrate the results of achieving these objectives.

PART III

THE LAUSON SYSTEM: CASE STUDIES

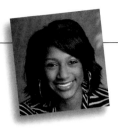

Comments Regarding
Cases Presented

A few comments regarding the cases presented are in order. This section is included because looking at patients' photos of actual treatment can convey a great deal of information. If a picture is worth a thousand words, the photos in this section speak volumes about the challenges and triumphs of The Lauson System's legion of "graduates." When it all comes down to it, the patient is the star of everything we do as orthodontists. His or her individual treatment reveals nuances that are impossible to share in any other way.

Orthodontists often talk about a "best age" to treat a patient. I think most would agree an optimal age range for the start of treatment is from ages eight to eleven. These young patients typically are very compliant and often even enthusiastic, which maximizes patient cooperation and thereby helps to achieve the best final result possible. Ideally, treatment is completed by the time a patient is a teenager. After all, at this time in their lives, they have other things they would rather be doing. If treatment hasn't been accomplished by then, Invisalign Teen may be a better option than braces. Nonetheless, the reality is that many patients are not able to begin treatment during the most optimal years. Rest assured, however, that even though this book is about the younger orthodontic patient, great results can be achieved with The Lauson System at any age, even including senior adults.

For ease of use, this section is divided into three chapters according to the ages of the patients, allowing the reader to zone in on the age group they are most interested in.

- Chapter 13 features preadolescent patients who started their treatment by age eight or nine. They had an early phase of treatment before all their permanent teeth had come in. These initial corrections allowed us to change the growth patterns for the better so that the final phase, to complete their treatment, more easily met the objectives of The Lauson System.
- Chapter 14 shows preteens who started their treatment at ages ten to twelve.
- Chapter 15 shows children who were in the teen years when having their treatment.

Cases presented are representative of the treatment results possible with the use of FFO and show very good results. However, not all cases yield the same successful results. Patient cooperation (or lack thereof) is always a strong determinant of any result when dealing with the human body. The removable treatment appliances that we recommend do require the patient to wear them full-time, as instructed. Educating the patient and the parents of treatment goals, along with emphasizing their imperative role in achieving those goals, leads to successful patient cooperation and a great result. These cases were challenging enough that the real power of FFO to treat without the need for surgery or extractions is evident.

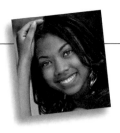

CHAPTER 13

Phase I
Treatment of Younger Patients
Cases 1-4

ll things being equal, the most ideal time to see a child contemplating orthodontic treatment is by age seven. By then the front teeth
are starting to come in and it is apparent where problems are appearing.
Crowding of teeth and overbites are already established and should ideally be
dealt with. Additionally, any adverse habits need to be addressed. Although
there is still plenty of time to address many things in a developing child,
the orthodontist has more flexibility and can better time treatment if the
child is evaluated before the issues become more full blown, and therefore,
more complex.

The patients in the following cases benefited from an early evaluation
and treatment as all cases were considered significantly complex. Less
complex cases can be postponed until around age ten. Because of the age of
the patients, the treatments were broken into Phase I treatment, followed by
a one to two year break, and then a one to two year Phase II treatment with
full braces once the remaining permanent teeth came in.

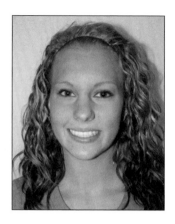

Case #1 – Alice

Alice was nearly eight years old when she came to our office for an evaluation. She had a substantial open bite in the front of her mouth (none of her front teeth touched) caused by a persistent anterior tongue posture and poor lip seal when swallowing. She also had moderate constriction of both her upper and lower dental arches, as well as moderately large tonsils. We recommended that Alice have her tonsils and adenoids evaluated for removal; this, however, did not occur until several years later when we further advised and she began oral myology therapy.

For some time, we worked with Alice to eliminate a forward-tongue posture without success, so the referral to the oral myologist gave her a number of one-on-one sessions of advanced therapy to eliminate the persistent habits. (In regards to working with a professional oral myologist or myofunctional therapist to complement treatment, it is vitally important that orthodontic treatment be performed without the hindrance of an adverse habit, which can make any result unstable, as discussed in Chapter 10. The necessity of a collaborative spirit among competent professionals to achieve great, long-term results cannot be overemphasized.)

We began our treatment with the use of upper and lower removable Schwarz appliances. What normally should take four to six months took much longer due to Alice not wearing the appliances as instructed during this phase. Eventually, however, our objectives were met. When the desired expansion was completed, we took a break for just a few months, and then placed the braces.

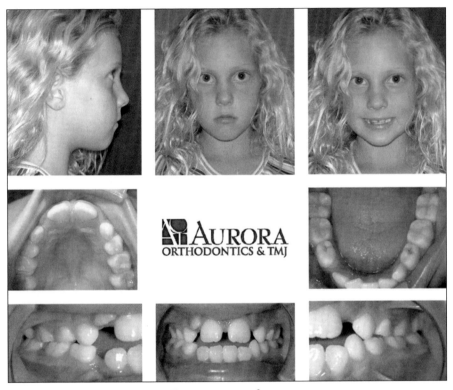

Pretreatment photos

Because of additional challenges with Alice's uncorrected tongue habit, progress was delayed by at least a year. I made the mistake with Alice, and several other patients along the way, of not demanding (early in treatment) that she see an oral myologist for help with her adverse tongue habit. Also, I should have insisted that the enlarged tonsils be removed earlier to help with the restricted airway issues that exacerbated the oral habits.

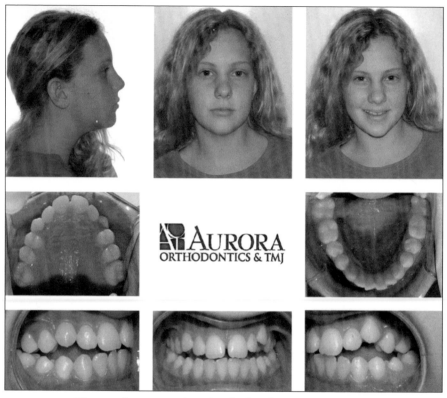

Photos after expansion, just before braces were placed

Many parents may be reluctant to follow through with extra expense items, such as these procedures, considering they are already paying for the orthodontics. However, all parents want the best for their children and if the doctor and staff properly explain the procedures, the extra expenses are usually not a problem. In spite of the delay with these procedures, this case turned out beautifully, even though it tested the collective patience of parents, child, and orthodontist along the way! All the struggles along the way were worth it to get such a great result for this beautiful, young lady. This is a case wherein a traditional approach to treatment would have either removed permanent teeth or used a surgical approach to close down the open bite. Note our final result, which avoided surgery and permanent tooth removal.

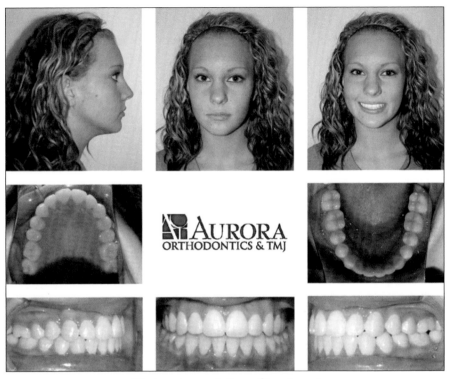

Photos at completion of treatment

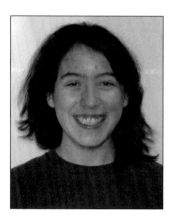

Case # 2 – Judy

When Judy came to our office, she was eight years old and still had a persistent thumb-sucking habit that had caused an open bite in the front teeth. Although most children will stop thumb sucking before they enter grade school, some continue with this destructive habit well past this age. Additionally, Judy had also acquired an anterior tongue-thrust habit. Because of these adverse habits, the lower jaw was retruded (Class II molar relationship) and the upper arch was severely constricted. This put the back teeth on the left into crossbite and caused the front teeth to protrude significantly, a condition known as overjet. The pretreatment pictures reveal a substantial distortion of the bone structure of the upper jaw caused by the persistent thumb habit and the tongue thrust.

Our treatment took into consideration the adverse oral habits of the thumb sucking and tongue thrust. We corrected the narrowness of the upper jaw and its relationship to the lower jaw. A modified, upper Schwarz appliance took care of these demands. We added a habit-correction device to the Schwarz as a reminder to Judy to keep her thumb out of her mouth and to keep her tongue properly positioned at the roof of her mouth. I'm happy to say this appliance was quite successful in accomplishing these goals. Then we went in a holding pattern, with Judy wearing the appliance just at night until all her permanent teeth came in.

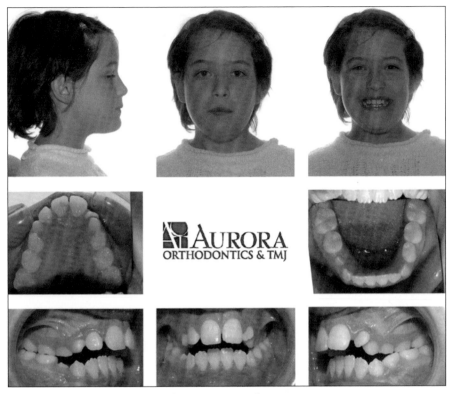

Pretreatment photos

When Judy was ten years old, she had braces placed. Her thumb habit was well behind her at this time, but her tongue-thrusting habit persisted. Because this would give Judy an incomplete result, which would not be stable, we referred her to an oral myologist who worked one-on-one with her in order to correct the tongue habit. As expected, this additional therapy was successful and twenty-two months later she was able to have her braces off, completing her treatment and achieving all nine keys to lower facial harmony.

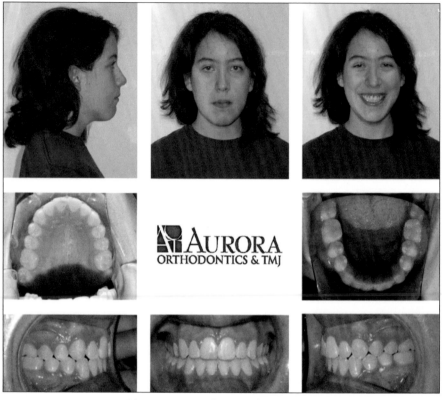

Photos at completion of treatment

Additional comments regarding Judy's treatment are as follows: The change in shape of the upper jaw was accomplished through FFO, resulting in a beautiful, broad smile.

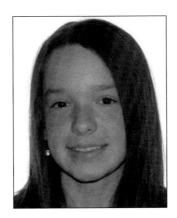

Case # 3 – Donna

Nine-year-old Donna came to my office after her dentist told her parents that there was no room in her mouth for many of her permanent teeth to come in later. This is a common problem for many children and a primary reason that parents seek orthodontic treatment for their children. In her case, traditional orthodontic treatment would likely have recommended the removal of up to four permanent bicuspid teeth in order to correct her bite.

Because Donna's upper jaw was very underdeveloped, I knew we had to enlarge it significantly. Consequently, I used a 3-way sagittal expansion appliance, the most powerful of the FFO appliances, on the upper arch. The lower arch, also constricted, was expanded with a lip bumper. We began treatment on her in spite of the fact that she didn't have many of her permanent teeth yet. There is a significant advantage to doing this type of treatment while many of the baby teeth are still present. During this time the permanent teeth are forming and coming into the mouth. If left to develop in a constricted jawbone, these teeth have to move significantly out of alignment even though they have not come into the mouth yet; in other words, the developing teeth are already crowded in the bone structure. Expanding the bone structure relieves the crowding, giving the teeth more room as they come into the mouth.

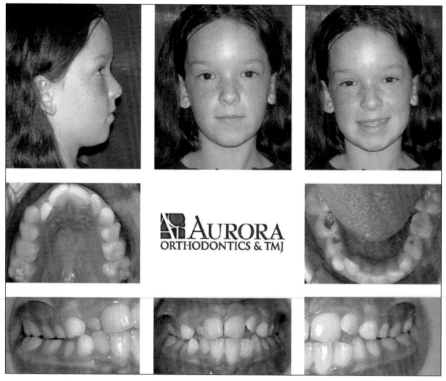

Pretreatment photos showing significant crowding of teeth

The photos below show the improvement after the initial phase of treatment, before braces were placed.

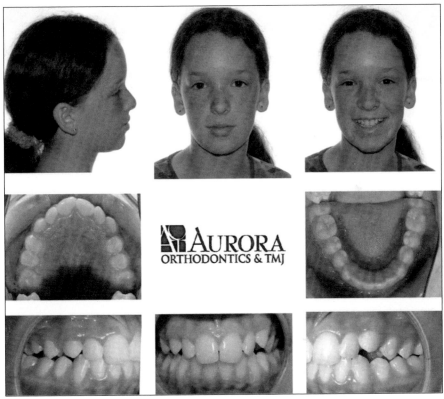

Photos after Phase I with FFO treatment

The remaining treatment occurred with braces once the rest of the baby teeth were gone and the new, permanent teeth came in. Because the initial treatment with orthopedic appliances had occurred, not too much was left to do except make sure all the permanent teeth were placed properly and that all functions were ideal. The treatment finished with a straightforward placement of braces. The following photos show Donna's final result.

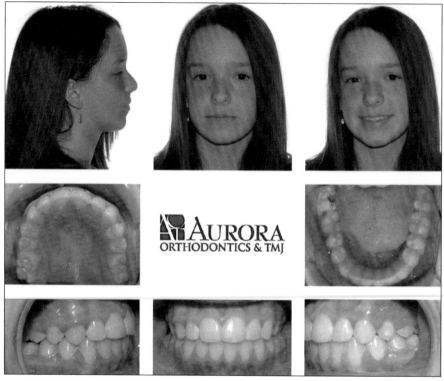

Photos at completion of treatment

Any patient or orthodontist would be very proud to show off these results. Had the initial phase not been completed properly, the work of getting all keys completed would have been more difficult at the time all permanent teeth had appeared.

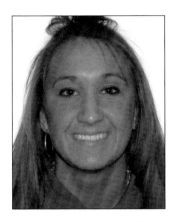

Case # 4 – Becky

Anine-year-old girl by the name of Becky came to me with a severely underdeveloped upper jaw, resulting in an underbite (skeletal Class III relationship). Seven of the nine keys to lower facial harmony were not present when she presented for treatment. These included nasal breathing obstruction, forward head posture, and TMJ clicking. As such, I knew our treatment should focus on achieving as many of these goals as possible in as short a time as possible—there was no time to waste.

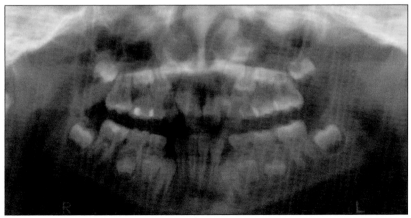

Panoramic x-ray showing severe upper crowding of teeth

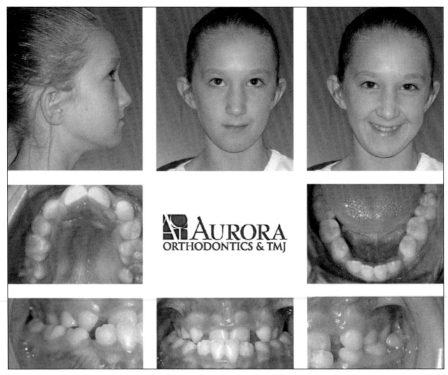

Pretreatment photos showing extreme upper crowding
and virtually all teeth in crossbite

Because the upper jaw was so underdeveloped, Becky had teeth growing on top of teeth high up in her bone structure. These were permanent teeth that had nowhere to go once they were developed and ready to come into her mouth. That is why it was so important to create new bone structure for these new teeth as soon as possible.

We used two different FFO appliances to stimulate new bone growth in her upper jaw. First, a 3-way sagittal appliance with posterior coverage was used to correct the crossbite. Once this was achieved, a Schwarz appliance was used to complete the remainder of the expansion needed on the upper jaw. Becky was very cooperative and voiced that she experienced almost no discomfort during the year or so of this phase of treatment. By the end of this first phase we had made great progress toward eliminating the problem areas discussed above.

We created much better lower-facial balance by developing considerably more bone structure in both the upper and lower jaws. Note the improvement in the areas around Becky's nose; she was able to breathe much easier through her nose and the TMJ clicking was no longer present. Becky's posture had improved, too, and her teeth crowding and crossbites were nearly eliminated as well.

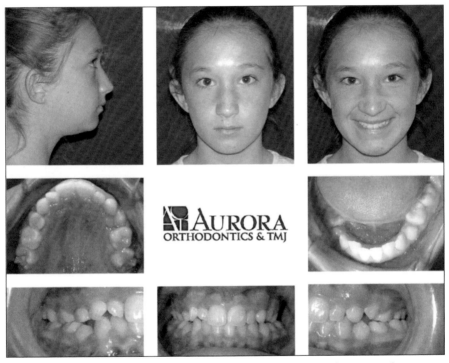

Photos taken after initial FFO phase showing crossbites mostly corrected for a much more manageable treatment in the future

All that was left to do was wait another year or so for the rest of Becky's permanent teeth to come in so that braces could be placed to complete treatment. During this time, retainers were worn to hold the teeth and expanded jaws. Once the remaining permanent teeth made an appearance, the second phase of treatment began with some additional expansion before braces were placed. The second phase of treatment, about fifteen months in total, yielded an excellent final result.

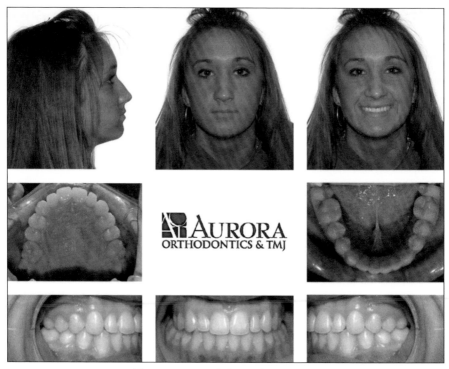

Photos at completion of treatment

Additional comments regarding Becky's treatment are as follows: A critical step toward a successful result is accomplished on the very first visit—this includes the evaluation, diagnosis, and treatment planning. We were able to achieve a beautiful result with Becky because we thoroughly evaluated the situation before we started the work. We knew what we needed to accomplish in order to have the best result and knew what could or could not be accomplished with the treatment appliances we chose to use.

Many practitioners using a more traditional orthodontic approach do not recognize the value in the use of the FFO treatment appliances used and therefore would not have been able to duplicate our results. Many don't believe treatment can be achieved without surgery. They believe that this type of skeletal problem can only be successfully resolved with a surgical approach when facial growth is completed in midteen years. At this time the surgery is performed to move the bones of the face into their proper place.

Another important observation needs to be made here. Surgeons are very good at taking away bone but less able to add more bone, so their surgical decisions may be based on that fact. Many surgically treated cases like Becky's incorrectly reduce the lower jaw to match a deficient upper jaw, producing an undesirable result—retrusion of both the upper and lower jaws, as well as other unintended consequences. Becky's case shows that excellent results can be achieved, including great facial balance, without surgery or removal of permanent teeth.

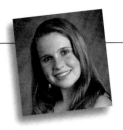

CHAPTER 14

Full Phase Treatment, Preteens
Cases 5-7

Children in adolescence present a very ideal age for treatment. If the orthodontic problem is not severe, it can be handled very nicely at this age. Patients typically are very cooperative and even enthusiastic about their treatment. After all, they are not teenagers yet. Therefore, we as orthodontists consider this an optimal time to treat most problems.

Skeletal growth problems, such as the very common narrow upper jaw, can best be handled before all the permanent teeth come in around age twelve. When FFO is handled at this time with an appliance such as a Schwarz, the bone is enlarged and can have a very positive effect on the eruption of teeth that may be developing crowded. Many apparent impacted cuspid teeth can actually start coming in much straighter once the bone structure is increased in size.

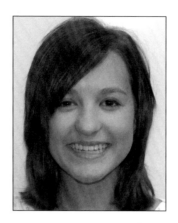

Case # 5 – Abby

At the time Abby came to our office for an initial evaluation, she was ten and a half years old. She had a slight underbite, with the upper front incisors hitting inside the lower incisors. She had severe dental crowding of her upper teeth, the result of a small upper jaw. Her lower jaw lacked the space to allow the teeth to come in straight, but it was not as far off as the upper jaw was.

She had moderately large tonsils and adenoids, and evidence of mouth breathing was present. Palpations of the muscles of the lower jaw, neck, and shoulders were done, as they should be in any initial evaluation to determine if there are any dysfunctions present within the patient's musculature.

For Abby, there was sensitivity in the lower jaw and neck muscles, an early warning sign for TMD. Also, Abby possessed a forward head posture caused by a too-far-back-functioning lower jaw. Over time, this posture could cause neck strain and a loss of the normal curvature in the neck, medically referred to as loss of cervical lordosis, which leads to a restriction of normal head and neck movements. (Please see more discussion on this very important subject in Chapter 8.)

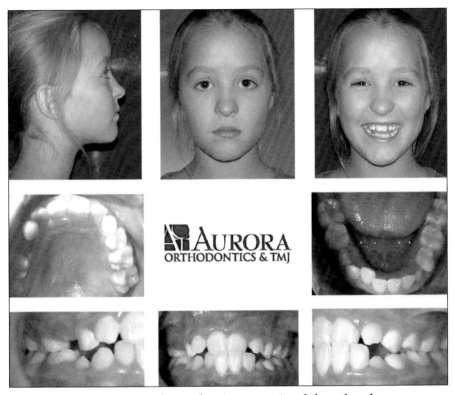

Pretreatment photos showing constricted dental arches

Both jaws needed expansion to achieve Key #1, a fully developed maxilla, as well as an ideal relationship to each other and to create room for the proper alignment of all the teeth. The mouth-breathing habit—which contributed to the dental malocclusion and played a significant role in Abby's poor head posture—needed to be stopped to achieve a stable result. We kept the moderately enlarged tonsils and adenoids (which did not have to be removed at this time) under a watchful eye. The removal of tonsils and adenoids could come later, if necessary. We made Abby's parents aware of our goals, which included elimination of the mouth-breathing habit.

We widened the upper jaw using a 3-way sagittal appliance and widened the dental arch form to match the upper by using a lip bumper. This eliminated the mouth-breathing habit and gained the ideal full arch forms necessary to straighten the teeth to an ideal result. The widening of the upper jaw took longer than normal—close to a year—and waiting on teeth to come in added some additional time for Abby to wear the upper appliance. Braces were placed for the last twenty-two months to complete our treatment. All treatment objectives were accomplished and the result below demonstrates that all nine keys were achieved.

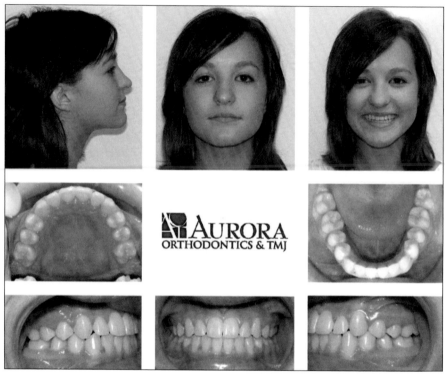

Photos at completion of treatment

Additional comments regarding Abby's treatment are as follows: The nine keys to lower facial harmony were achieved with a quite straightforward approach. I remember my days as a beginning orthodontist, before discovering these FFO techniques; I used to struggle to find the right answers for this type of patient. Would I extract teeth, or would I try to shoehorn everything in knowing that my result may not be stable? Would I wait till growth was more complete to know what I was dealing with? Those types of questions don't haunt me anymore, as I know that I can alter or enhance growth with this type of treatment. The bigger truth is that with FFO we can create new bone structure at any time during life, even in an individual whose growth is complete.

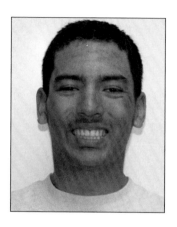

Case # 6 – David

D avid was twelve and a half years old when he came to our office as a new patient. With an eleven millimeter overjet and front teeth protruding, his condition was considered an extreme skeletal discrepancy. His bite on the left side was considerably off with the molars in crossbite and in a full Class II molar relationship (see Chapter 6). Both dental arches were constricted, but the upper was more extreme. His tonsils were moderate in size.

As a result of his reduced ability to breathe through his nose, he had acquired the undesirable habit of mouth breathing. With some encourage-ment and coaching, this habit could be controlled with a little concentration on David's part. However, I knew that when we expanded his upper jaw, his ability to breathe through his nose would greatly increase. His jaw joints checked out normally, but he did have some tenderness in his neck muscles as a result of a forward head posture.

We began treatment with a Schwarz expander in the upper arch and four months later added a lower Schwarz to help his lower jaw relate to the expanded upper arch. Patient cooperation was not stellar, and it took us a year to get enough expansion to place braces. Like many boys his age, David was also not on good terms with the rubber bands we required him to wear during the braces phase. However, we did eventually reach the goal. The synergy between the patient, his parents, and our office was critical, and it was important in this case to go the extra mile, especially since David was really trying to do his job.

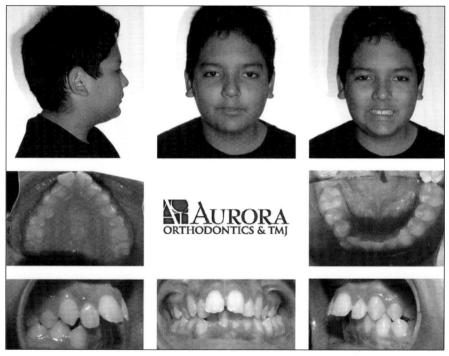

Pretreatment photos showing extreme overbite and narrow arches

In addition to the previous concerns, David developed a poor tongue-posture habit that needed to be addressed, necessitating a referral to an oral myologist for individual sessions. The nine keys were achieved in the end and the braces were removed after two and a half years of treatment.

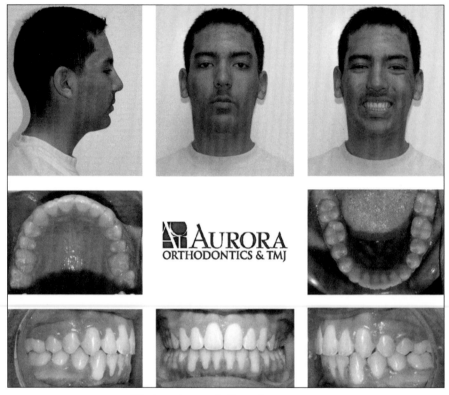

Photos at completion of treatment

Additional comments regarding David's treatment are as follows: In spite of the fact that treatment took longer than expected, we did achieve a very good result and David and his parents were delighted with his handsome smile.

A traditional treatment argument could have been made to remove four bicuspid teeth and do orthodontic treatment. This patient was much better off keeping all of his permanent teeth and ended up with a broad, confident smile.

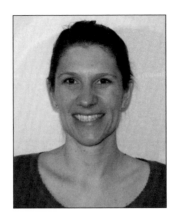

Case #7 – Sandy

Encouraged by an article I had written for a local community news-paper entitled "Dentofacial Orthopedics, A Treatment Whose Time Has Come," twelve-year-old Sandy's mother called our office in June of 1991. Sandy's orthodontist had recently recommended surgery—involving breaking and resetting the jaw, followed by braces when her daughter turned sixteen. My article, which detailed the innovative methods we used in our office that eliminated the need for tooth extraction and surgery (whereas traditional orthodontic methods required one or both), gave the distraught mother hope. "All I want for Sandy is straight teeth, hopefully without pulling teeth and without surgery," she confided to me, to which I could only smilingly respond, "You've come to the right place!"

Initial evaluation of my soon-to-be new patient revealed, among other findings, a substantial underbite. Dentists call this condition a bilateral posterior crossbite along with an anterior crossbite. In other words, all the teeth in the upper jaw were on the inside of the teeth in the lower jaw. The upper jaw was substantially constricted, causing significant crowding of her upper teeth, while there was almost no crowding on the lower teeth. I could see that there was what doctors call a midface deficiency and maxillary hypoplasia (skeletal Class III relationship). In layman's terms, this meant that there was a substantial deficiency of growth of the upper jaw area,

137

which resulted in a lack of support for the upper lips and the nose, as seen in the before pictures below. Sandy also had an anterior tongue thrust (see Chapter 11), which was likely due to the small size of the upper jaw and the lack of space for her tongue to be in the normal position at the roof of her mouth. She also had pain and clicking in her right TMJ. The x-rays revealed that the right jaw joint was out of proper alignment.

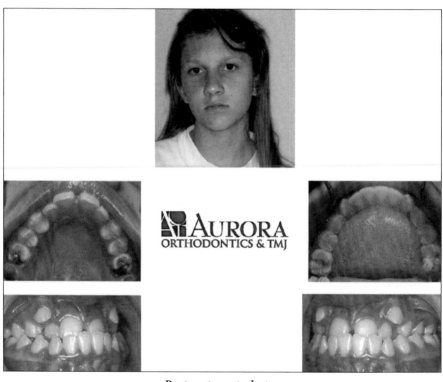

Pretreatment photos

The traditional approach (as described before) has long been, and continues to be, to wait until growth is complete, around age sixteen for young ladies. In Sandy's case, this meant surgery on the lower jaw to reduce its prominence, the extraction of at least two bicuspid teeth, and then straightening the teeth with braces. This traditional approach would have involved unnecessary surgery and extraction of permanent teeth, invariably causing a poor treatment result.

The problem was not the lower-jaw protrusion, but the inadequate development of the upper jaw. Realizing I needed the use of a powerful FFO appliance for this correction, I used an upper 3-way sagittal appliance for the initial phase of Sandy's treatment. This was necessary to expand and enlarge the entire bone structure of the upper jaw to bring it into balance with the lower jaw. I also wanted to gain a normal TMJ function during this time. This phase was accomplished within a nine-month period. The photos below were taken on the day Sandy's braces were placed.

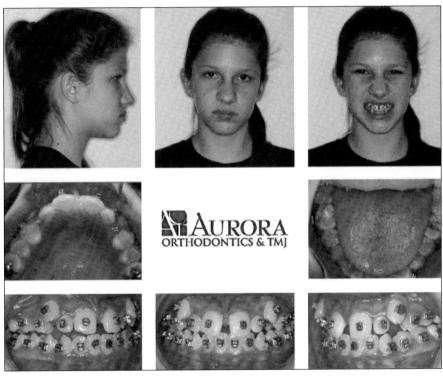

Photos after initial phase treatment, just after braces were placed, showing correction of crossbites and enlargement of upper jaw

As you can see, with the upper arch expanded, the teeth were in a much better position to straighten with traditional braces.

The key here is to understand that without the FFO phase, this treatment would not have been possible, and Sandy would have had to face the surgery and permanent teeth removal her mother so badly feared. Below is our final result. Note the improvement in facial contours, especially in the upper lip and nose area.

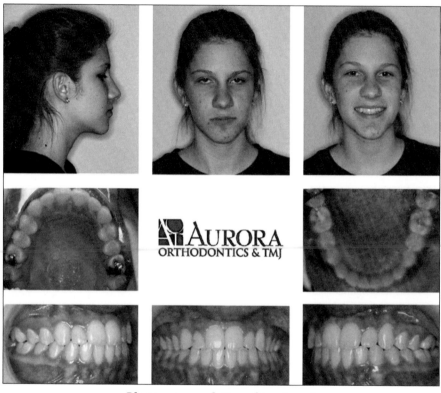

Photos at completion of treatment

In preparation for this book, we contacted Sandy and asked her to come into my office. She happily obliged, and the updated photos of her show that the results were still very stable seventeen years after treatment was completed.

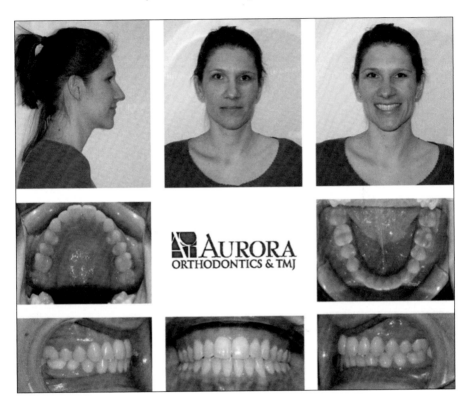

Now thirty-one years old, here is a candid, funny, and enlightening testimonial about her treatment:

I was pretty young when my parents started consulting orthodontists about my teeth, probably eleven or twelve. I remember a visit to one office, and the orthodontist recommended surgically 'breaking' my jaw and resetting it to fix my problem. I believe it would have required having my mouth wired shut for six weeks. I was terrified at the possibility, especially at such a young age. My parents, of course, wanted a treatment option that didn't involve surgery. Throughout middle school, I rarely smiled because I was so self-conscious about my teeth. My braces were removed when I was in the ninth grade. I remember going to church with my family shortly after having my braces removed. I had only been there a few minutes when someone commented with surprise, 'She's smiling!' For the first time ever, I felt like I had a pretty smile! It has been over sixteen years since my treatment ended and I still feel like I have a pretty smile. My treatment with Dr. Lauson was effective and still is to this day. It was worth every second with metal in my mouth!

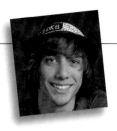

CHAPTER 15

Full Phase Treatment, Teens Cases 8-10

Treatment during the teenage years sometimes presents some special challenges. Many orthodontic problems are already corrected by this time. This is because the twelve-year molars are usually in and orthodontic treatment may already be completed. Social and hormonal changes are taking place in the teen and his or her attention to things the parent's desire is waning. "Braces are for kids, but teens prefer Invisalign" is a very true statement and one of the reasons Invisalign Teen is really taking off. However, I just really got into Invisalign Teen treatment within the last year, so I am not presenting treated cases in this section, but I did so at the end of Chapter 12. Teenage patients are considered by many orthodontists to be treated like adults, since most facial growth (especially in girls) is nearing completion. Fortunately, ideal FFO treatment can still be accomplished, as it can at any age, with good patient cooperation. The following cases exhibit what is routinely accomplished.

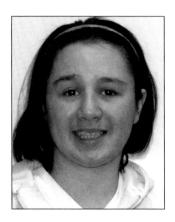

Case # 8 – Vanessa

Vanessa, the older sister of Jake (who we met at the end of Chapter 6), came to our office at the age of thirteen. The examination revealed that her most significant problem was very narrow, underdeveloped dental arches and severe crowding of the teeth as a result. She was also a mouth breather and had beginning symptoms of TMD. Even with great patient cooperation, Vanessa's situation would be challenging to treat.

As a special-needs patient, initially we had concern regarding her ability to understand and comply with our treatment recommendations. At the consultation appointment, extensive discussions with Vanessa's parents about our recommendations and concerns revealed that they understood the challenge and that they really wanted the best for their daughter.

During that meeting we discussed three different options: Option #1—certainly the best, if it could be accomplished—was to expand the dental arches to an ideal form and then straighten the teeth with braces. Our concern was that Vanessa might not adapt to the recommended removable orthopedic appliances, which she would have to wear at all times (including mealtimes), only taking them out to brush and clean her teeth. Option #2 was to do a more traditional orthodontic approach and remove all four first-bicuspid teeth and follow with braces. The advantage of this was that Vanessa's cooperation would not be as critical, since the braces would be fixed on the teeth and there would be nothing to take out of her mouth. Option #3 was to do nothing and wait until Vanessa gained more maturity.

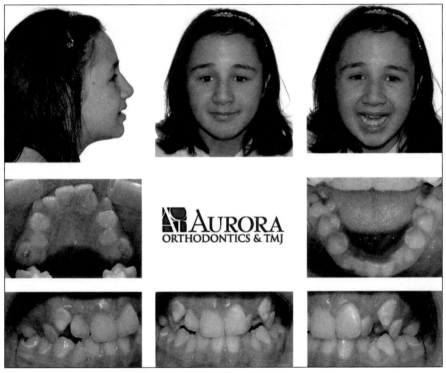

Pretreatment photos showing extreme crowding and narrow arches

After much deliberation, which included discussions with Vanessa, those involved decided on option #1. Why not go for the most ideal result, despite the potential challenges along the way? A huge factor in our favor was that her younger brother was just beginning treatment, too, and he also needed to wear removable expansion appliances. While Jake was not a special-needs patient and his situation was not as challenging as his big sister's, we counted on Vanessa's encouragement that her little brother was going through the same process. By the same token, if she didn't have the treatment, she would have been very disappointed and may have felt left behind. Luckily, Vanessa understood that her teeth were very crooked, and at the end of the day she genuinely wanted to have the treatment. Encouraged by my kind and gentle staff, she felt she could do it and knew we would always be there to help her, if necessary. In a word, Vanessa was a real trooper.

When we began treatment for Vanessa, she was just a couple months past her thirteenth birthday. We used upper and lower Schwarz appliances to develop and expand both upper and lower jaws and dental arches. All went well with the upper Schwarz appliance, but difficulties with the lower appliance caused us to shift gears and go with a fixed lower E-Arch (see Appendix A for description of all treatment appliances), also known as an Arnold expander. Fortunately, the upper arch required the most work, and the lower arch was less critical.

As a general rule, once the upper jaw is expanded appropriately (which is truly an increase of bone size), the lower can be expanded much easier. Using slow palatal expansion on the upper arch we were able to stimulate bone growth, eliminating the need to extract any permanent teeth and to create a beautiful, full smile.

The lower expansion is predominately uprighting of lower teeth that have tipped inward following a narrow upper arch. With the E-Arch we were able to get the necessary expansion on the lower jaw, and since Vanessa did quite well with the upper Schwarz, expansion was accomplished in the next nine months. So, nine months out, we placed the braces on Vanessa. Sixteen months later, we removed the braces and completed this nonextraction treatment over a twenty-five month period. We resolved the TMD and Vanessa breathed through her nose with ease. The following pictures show the happy end result.

Additional comments regarding Vanessa's treatment are as follows: Giving the parents and child three viable treatment options allowed them to make an informed decision based on the successful treatment of many thousands of other patients with this method. Despite the inherent challenges of working with a special-needs patient, success was all but assured because a great deal of compassion, understanding, and cooperation existed between my team and the family.

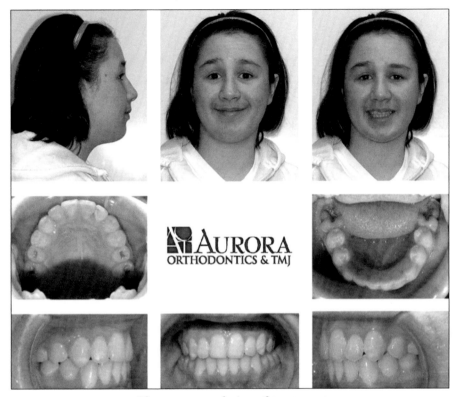

Photos at completion of treatment

With a traditional approach it is likely that Vanessa would have had four permanent bicuspid teeth removed to achieve straight teeth. Unfortunately, this would have resulted in not only a smaller smile with four fewer teeth, but also the TMD may have gotten worse over time. The mouth breathing that had occurred prior to treatment may not have been resolved and may have led to many of the dysfunctions listed in Chapter 5. All objectives of the nine keys to lower facial harmony were achieved with our treatment.

There are valuable lessons to be learned from this case:

First, we should watch not to prejudge a patient's ability to cooperate during treatment. The patient's personal motivation and family support are very big factors in treatment success. Professionals should always work to help create a better understanding of the work that needs to be done and what is expected of the patient and family. Patient education is very important.

Second, practices can consistently get a 95% compliance rate with patients wearing FFO appliances if proper patient education and motivation are used. This case proves that if a special-needs patient, like Vanessa, can successfully wear her removable treatment appliances, anyone needing them can do likewise given the proper instruction and motivation. Orthodontists and dentists doing orthodontics need to get past the idea that their patients won't wear the FFO appliances—a myth belied by the willingness of highly motivated Invisalign patients to wear the aligners to achieve the desired results.

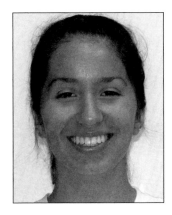

Case # 9 – Barbara

When Barbara, fourteen, first came to my office for an evaluation, she had narrow jaws and cuspid teeth that were completely blocked out by their neighboring teeth, so they couldn't come in.

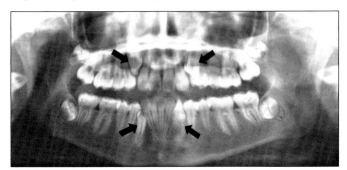

Pretreatment panoramic x-ray showing blocked-out cuspid teeth

To compound the problem, Barbara also had a clicking jaw joint (TMJ) on her right side. This occurred because the lower jaw was getting trapped behind the constricted upper teeth and jaw, causing the lower jaw to retrude too far and resulting in the jaw joint getting out of alignment. We began treatment by widening the upper jaw to a more ideal arch form, which accomplished two things: First, it created much more room for the blocked-out canine teeth, therefore allowing the braces to do the remaining work. Second, a wider upper arch also released the trapped lower jaw, allowing it to come more forward, correcting the dysfunctional TMJ. Correcting these problems early helped to prevent future functional problems with the TMJ.

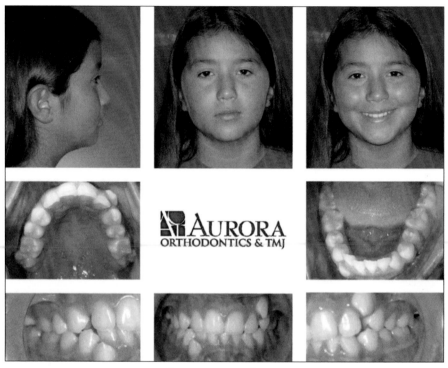

Pretreatment photos

A side note: a mistake often made during orthodontic treatment is not taking seriously the clicking jaw joint. Unfortunately, there is a lack of training given in dental schools in this area. Unless the dentist doing orthodontics takes much further training in this area, he or she won't have the ability to adequately address the problem of TMD. As with any medical concern, early detection of TMJ dysfunctions can prevent a host of unpleasant problems in a child's future.

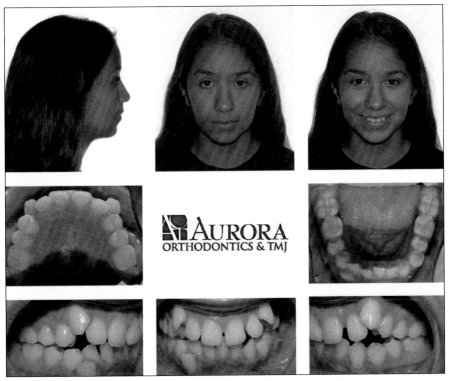

Photos after FFO expansion phase, just before braces were placed

Even though the expansion appliances had done their work and we were ready for Barbara's braces, the expansion was held for another two full months. This additional period, which allowed for the bones to become more solid and therefore more stable, was critical to hold the change. Fortunately, this didn't delay treatment. Braces were placed and the continued wearing of the expansion appliances helped to maintain the new bone structure. (At first, a patient may not think this is fair—having to wear both the expander and braces at the same time—but when he or she realizes that it can cut two months off of treatment time by doing both at once, no one ever objects.)

The support of the continued wearing of the expander and the progression into heavier arch wires that held the expanded arch form created better stability of the expansion. In the final phase, the braces were worn for about fifteen months (an average time). The following are pictures of Barbara's final result.

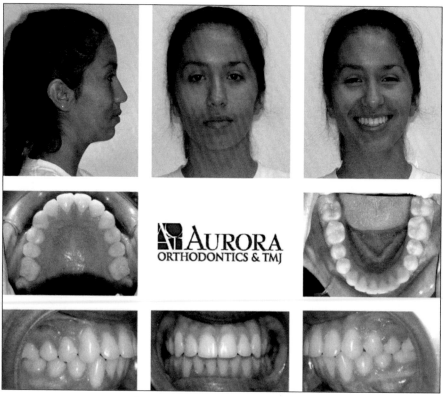

Photos at completion of treatment

Additional comments regarding Barbara's treatment are as follows: Critical steps toward a successful result, including evaluation, diagnosis, and treatment planning, were accomplished on the very first visit. We were able to achieve a beautiful result with Barbara because we thoroughly evaluated the situation before we started the work. We knew what we needed to accomplish in order to have the best result and knew what could or could not be accomplished with the treatment appliances we chose to use. Many practitioners using a more traditional orthodontic approach do not recognize the value in the use of the FFO treatment appliances and, therefore, would likely have removed four bicuspid teeth to straighten the remaining ones. This would have left the narrow arch forms, and the treatment may have contributed to future TMJ problems.

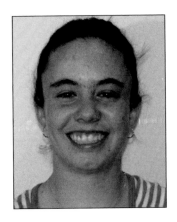

Case #10 – Roxanne

When we first saw thirteen-year-old Roxanne at her initial examination, we observed a very common problem: narrow arch forms with significant dental crowding. The upper cuspid teeth, being the last teeth to come in, were blocked out and stuck out like fangs. This commonly occurs when Class II molar relationships exist and the upper jaw is underdeveloped. The lower front teeth had moderate crowding. Other findings were as follows: enlarged tonsils and adenoids; clicking in her right TMJ; tenderness on palpation of numerous jaw and neck muscles; loss of cervical lordosis (loss of normal neck curvature). Additionally, the adverse oral habits of mouth breathing and night teeth grinding (known as bruxism) were present. This was a case where traditional orthodontic treatment might have called for removing four bicuspid teeth, perhaps leaving the aforementioned problems uncorrected.

Although our plan was to expand the upper and lower arches, we wanted to address the mouth-breathing problem, so we referred Roxanne to an otolaryngology specialist for an evaluation of the enlarged tonsils and adenoids, which were found to be obstructive and were removed without incident. We also gave Roxanne nasal breathing exercises to get rid of the bad habit of mouth breathing.

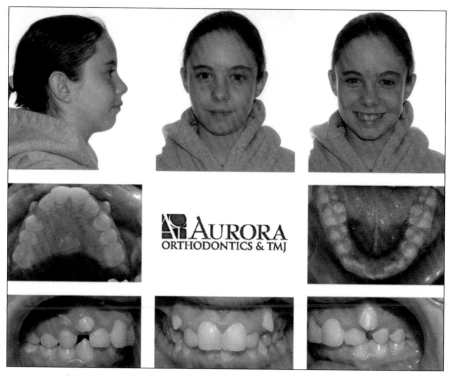

Pretreatment photos showing crowding and narrow arches

For our treatment, we used an upper 3-way sagittal appliance with an anterior bite plate and a lower Schwarz expansion appliance. With good patient cooperation we achieved our objectives within four months, and braces were placed. After another fifteen months of braces, Roxanne's treatment was complete, achieving all objectives of the nine keys to lower facial harmony.

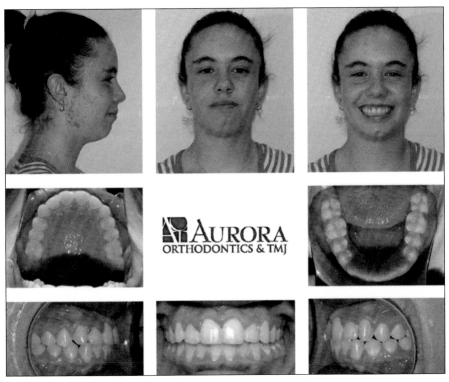

Photos at completion of treatment

Appendixes

The following appendixes are meant to give the reader additional details to further enhance his or her understanding of the treatment recommended. Appendix A shows pictures and descriptions of the treatment appliances used to accomplish the desired result. Appendix B includes some articles that talk about the philosophies of the treatment used. This will help the reader to understand the invaluable benefit that early intervention can have to prevent some very debilitating conditions in the future. Finally, Appendix C is meant to give many fellow professionals a further understanding of the ideas presented herein. These may be written for the dental and medical community, but the general public will also gain valuable information, should they so desire to plunge in.

APPENDIX A: TREATMENT APPLIANCES

1. Simple Expansion Appliances

   a. Schwarz Expansion Appliance

   b. Lower Schwarz (or Jackson) Expansion Appliance

   c. Quad Helix Expansion Appliance

   d. Hyrax Expansion (or Rapid Palatal Expander) Appliance

   e. E-Arch Expansion Appliance

   f. Lip Bumper

2. Complex Expansion Appliances

    a. 2-Way Sagittal Appliance

    b. 3-Way Sagittal Appliance

    c. V-Expansion Appliance

    d. Twin Block Appliance

3. Bite Plates

    a. Anterior Bite Plate

    b. Anterior Bite Ramp

    c. Posterior Bite Plate

    d. Mandibular Orthotic

4. Types of Braces

    a. Traditional Metal Braces

    b. Ceramic or Clear Braces

    c. Invisalign® or Other Aligners

5. Retainers

    a. Hawley Retainer

    b. Invisible Retainer

    c. Fixed Retainers

    d. Tooth Positioner

APPENDIX B: PERTINENT ARTICLES AND BLOGS

1. "ADHD and Sleep Disorders" – WebMD Article

2. "Parkinson's Disease and TMJ Dysfunction: A Mysterious Connection" – AOTMJ Blog

3. "Megatrends in Orthodontics" – AOTMJ Blog

4. "Protandim, a Breakthrough Anti-aging and Health Product" – AOTMJ Blog

APPENDIX C: FOR DENTAL AND MEDICAL PROFESSIONALS

1. "A New Gold Standard for Orthodontic Evaluations" – Article

2. Dr. Lauson's Review of Book: *Epigenetic Orthodontics in Adults*

3. "In Search of Improved Skeletal Transverse Diagnosis" – Article

4. "The Occlusal-TMJ-Cervical Connection" – Paper and Chart

5. Excerpt from *Orthodontics for the TMJ/TMD Patient*

6. Symptoms Rating Sheet

7. Nasopharyngeal Obstruction Chart

APPENDIX A

Treatment Appliances

The following are pictures of treatment appliances used with The Lauson System and an explanation of uses for each.

1. SIMPLE EXPANSION APPLIANCES

a. Schwarz Expansion Appliance

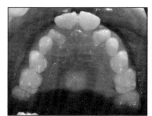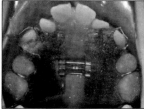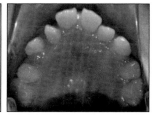

Before   *After expansion with Schwarz*   *After*

This removable treatment appliance is the simplest, most widely used, and most valuable of all orthopedic treatment appliances. It is used on the roof of the mouth to essentially push outward on the palate to increase bone structure on a patient whose upper jaw is narrow. It has a screw placed in its middle at the midpalatal suture. This screw is activated, or turned a quarter of a revolution, by a parent (or adult patient) about every two to three days. Over a four- to six-month period, the Schwarz appliance can achieve four to eight millimeters of expansion. For expansion beyond eight millimeters, the expansion screw is replaced and activation is resumed for the additional expansion required. This is possible because the midpalatal suture does not fuse at any time throughout life. Many times the Schwarz appliance is used in combination with a bite plate to accomplish two objectives at once. This appliance is ideal for patients who have developed the maturity (typically by age nine or above) to handle the responsibility of a removable appliance. It is also primarily used in cases that present mild to moderate crowding.

   b.   Lower Schwarz (or Jackson) Expansion Appliance

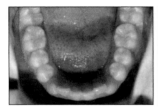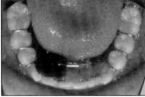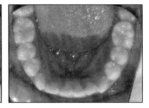

Before   *After expansion with Schwarz appliance*   *After*

The lower Schwarz appliance is a removable appliance with a screw in its center that is placed on the lower teeth. It extends lower to touch against the gums and below. The primary purpose of this appliance is to upright lower teeth that have been leaning inward to accommodate a small upper jaw. Some increase of bone structure occurs, as well, when the bone is pushed outward. Activations usually occur every three days; over a four-month period, two to four millimeters of expansion can be accomplished. This appliance is primarily used for patients nine years and older.

   c.   Quad Helix Expansion Appliance

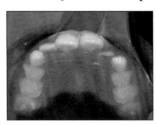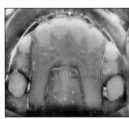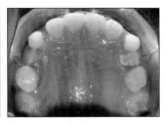

Before   *After expansion with Quad Helix*   *After*

The quad helix is an appliance that fits near the roof of the mouth and is fixed with orthodontic bands on the upper primary second-molar teeth. It uses a series of looped wires that spring outward with gentle pressure to create bone changes over a number of months. It is used on younger patients, typically ages six to nine, when cooperation with a removable appliance may be an issue. The doctor activates this appliance at the initial appointment when it is cemented into place. This appliance is not recommended for use with adult teeth due to the pressure applied directly to the teeth, which can result in tipping of teeth. It is for this reason that baby teeth are utilized while they are still present.

   d.   Hyrax Expansion (or Rapid Palatal Expander: RPE) Appliance

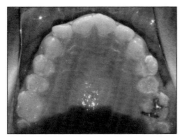 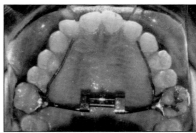

Before   *After expansion with Hyrax appliance*

The Hyrax appliance is generally used on older patients, ages nine and above, who are noncompliant with removable (Schwarz or sagittal) appliances. Because this appliance is usually fixed to the upper first-molar teeth, there is a limitation on how much expansion can be safely accomplished. Note in the picture above how much expansion has occurred at the first molars, but not at the other teeth. We advocate expansion with no more than one activation every third day, which is a much slower schedule than is generally recommended in traditional orthodontics. In fact, this appliance is commonly called a rapid palate expander (RPE) due to the frequency of activation in traditional orthodontics. Palatal suture release techniques are also recommended with this appliance.

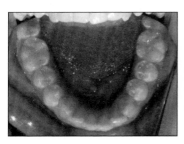 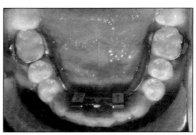

Before   *After expansion with Hyrax appliance*

This Hyrax expansion appliance used on the lower jaw performs in the same manner as the appliance on the upper jaw. It serves to help upright the lower teeth that have tipped in accommodating to a narrow upper arch. The same inherent concerns apply as with the upper RPE expanders.

e. E-Arch Expansion Appliance

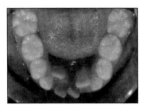 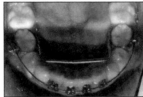 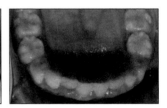

Before   *After expansion with E-Arch*   *After*

The E-arch is a valuable arch-development appliance used for the lower teeth and bone structure. It is fixed to the lower primary-second molars and consists of a spring-loaded wire on the inside of the teeth that gently pushes outward. Over about a six- to nine-month period, the arch gradually widens and results in more room for teeth. It is used for younger patients (six to nine years) when cooperation may be a concern due to immaturity.

f. Lip Bumper

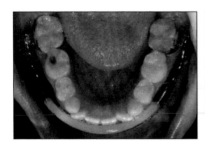 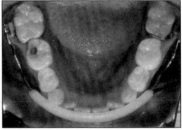

Before with Lip Bumper   *After expansion with Lip Bumper*

Where lower crowding is present, the lip bumper is a valuable treatment device that works the opposite way of most orthopedic treatment appliances. Instead of pushing outward on bone structure to create new bone, this innovative appliance works to stop the inward pressure, which tends to hold back growth. This creates an imbalance of the pressures (pressures in versus pressures out). Therefore, the bone expands in a very natural way. Although this method is slower than the more active "push" approach, there are other benefits in certain applications, such as holding back lower first molars while the lower second-bicuspid teeth erupt. Seven to eleven years of age is the appropriate range for use of this appliance; however, it should not be used once the primary second molars are gone.

2. COMPLEX EXPANSION APPLIANCES

a. 2-Way Sagittal Appliance

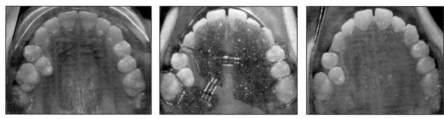

Before   *After expansion with 2-way sagittal*   *After*

A 2-way sagittal appliance, like a Schwarz appliance, widens the upper jaw. It is very effective when more extensive crowding or lack of bone struc-ture on one side of the mouth warrants the use of a second screw to develop more bone structure. Many times upper canine teeth are blocked out since these are the last teeth to come into the mouth. By that time, the space may already be gone. The 2-way sagittal appliance increases the bone structure in a front-to-back relationship on the side in which the second screw is used. In this example, the bicuspid tooth is blocked out before treatment.

b. 3-Way Sagittal Appliance

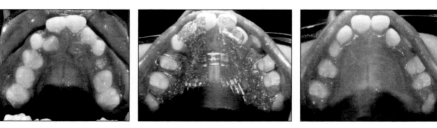

Before   *After expansion with 3-way sagittal*   *After*

In my opinion, the 3-way sagittal appliance is the most powerful ortho-pedic appliance in existence. This appliance is truly a game changer for a patient who has been told that he or she needs surgery due to an underde-veloped upper jaw. Just like the 2-way sagittal appliance, the 3-way sagittal appliance is used to create, as well as widen, bone structure in a front-to-back relationship, but this time on both sides. This appliance is used when there is a massive amount of crowding. Traditional orthodontists typically resort to extracting four bicuspid teeth to complete their patients' treatments. Without this marvelous appliance, surgery is certainly required to get the job done. The 3-way sagittal appliance, when properly worn, eliminates all of those discussions.

c.   V-Expansion Appliance

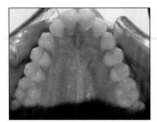 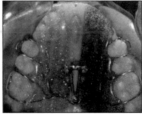 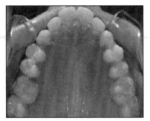

Before   *After expansion with V-expander*   *After*

The V-expansion appliance is used in a similar situation to the upper Schwarz appliance, with one primary exception: Sometimes the upper arch is fully expanded in the molar region. When this is the case, and no further expansion with the very back teeth is desirable, then the V-expan-sion appliance is perfect. This appliance works similarly to the Schwarz in that there are two halves with a screw in the center, but this is where the similarity ends. The V-expansion screw is put in at the back (posterior) of the appliance and opens like a fan when activated. So instead of an even pressure outward as in the Schwarz appliance, the V-expansion appliance moves only the front portion outward as the appliance is activated, and the back teeth remain in the same position. The result is that the V-shaped dental arch becomes a much fuller U-shaped dental arch, creating a full, celebrity-like smile.

d. Twin Block Appliance

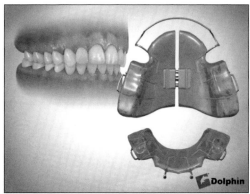

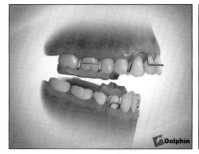
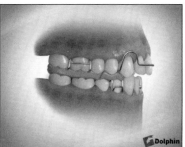

Illustrations courtesy Dolphin® Imaging & Management Solutions

The twin block appliance is used to correct a situation where the lower jaw is set too far back (retruded). It simultaneously works with the type of expansion screws found in a Schwarz or sagittal appliance to develop the full arch forms while the lower jaw is being corrected. These are used primarily on extreme cases since using a bite plate or bite ramp, although not as powerful, can accomplish a lesser but similar result.

3. BITE PLATES

a. Anterior Bite Plate

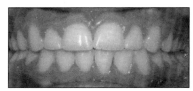
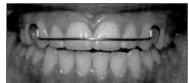

Without bite plate *With bite plate in place*

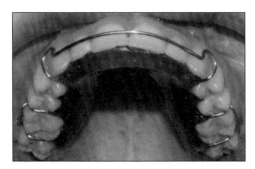

Picture shows thickness of acrylic
behind upper front teeth

The anterior bite plate, by itself or in combination with a Schwarz or sagittal appliance, can be very powerful in correcting overbites and "untrapping" the lower jaw so it can move forward into a more ideal position. It consists of a thickness of plastic placed behind the front teeth of the upper jaw. When the patient bites down, the lower front teeth come into contact with the plastic, thereby preventing the back teeth from touching. The patient is instructed to wear the appliance when eating, which allows the back teeth to grow in more, resulting in the correction of an overbite. The pictures above show the change after a Schwarz expander with an anterior bite plate is used.

b.   Anterior Bite Ramp

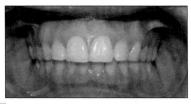
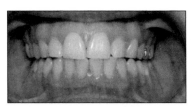

Without bite ramp   *With bite ramp in place*

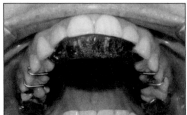
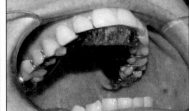

Pictures showing acrylic ramp

The anterior bite ramp is like an anterior bite plate, except that its purpose is to guide the lower jaw to a specific place, usually a forward position. This device is commonly used in combination with other types of appliances, including Hawley retainers, to correct an instance where an overbite may be returning or the lower jaw may be sliding back into a more retruded position.

    c.   Posterior Bite Plate

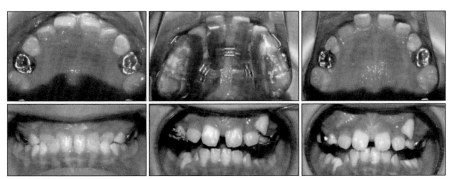

Before   *After expansion with posterior*   *After*
bite plate with 3-way sagittal

The posterior bite plate is a piece of plastic that fits over the back teeth and is usually an extension of another appliance like a Schwarz or a sagittal. When correcting teeth in crossbite, this is generally used to prop open the mouth to allow movement of the front teeth. Once the correction is made, the posterior bite plate is usually eliminated so that an ideal bite can be achieved.

    d.   Mandibular Orthotic

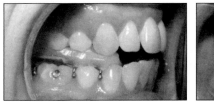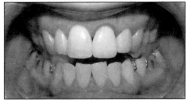

Pictures showing orthotic in place

In general, an orthotic is a device designed to support weak or ineffective joints and muscles. The orthotic used in my treatment is not to be confused with the type of orthotic used in your shoes! It is an appliance worn full-time in the mouth to reposition the lower jaw into a more ideal position. A sophisticated computer scan that tracks the movements of the jaw is used to put the jaw joint and facial muscles into a neuromuscularly balanced position that allows for healing in the area. In positioning the orthotic, we use electrotherapeutics (gentle electrical muscle and nerve stimulation to calm the muscles of the lower jaw). This allows healing to occur and reduces or eliminates most symptoms caused by TMD. This device is used in the first phase of treatment to correct the misalignment of the jaw joints. It is also worn during an additional phase of orthodontic treatment to correct the bite and bring it into alignment with the healthy position of the jaw joint.

4. TYPES OF BRACES

a. Traditional Metal Braces

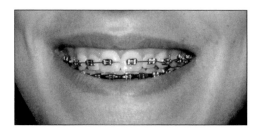

Traditional metal braces have been around for over a hundred years. It used to be that these braces were made to attach to bands that were fitted individually to each tooth. This tedious process literally took several hours and a couple appointments (lasting several hours each) for the orthodontist to complete. Today, with the newer, direct-bonded approach, braces are typically placed in about an hour. These metal braces are made of stainless steel and are much less bulky in the mouth than their predecessors. For those that have sensitivity to nickel, contemporary metal braces are also available in hypoallergenic metals, such as gold and titanium. Advancements in design have allowed for much of the treatment to be built into the braces themselves. That is because the individual braces have what is called torque and tip (or angulation) built into the slot of each bracket. These help to rotate and angle the teeth without having to put bends in the arch wire to achieve these movements. The "straight wire appliance," developed in the 1970s, is the preferred type of brace with many variations because it efficiently moves each tooth and consistently creates better results. With this appliance, every tooth has a different formula, thereby allowing each tooth to be positioned to its individual, ideal position. At the end of treatment a straight wire can then be used to finalize treatment results.

   b.   Ceramic or Clear Braces

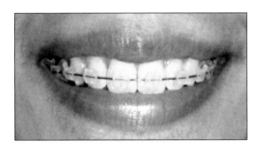

Clear braces were designed to address the adult patient's desire for a less obvious option to metal braces. Clear braces have been around for some time, at least since the 1970s. We started out primarily using plastic braces, but found them too weak to withstand the pressures needed to effectively move teeth. Ceramic braces—yes, you read that right, ceramic, much like the heat-hardened material that is your coffee cup—were developed as a better option in later years. Today the ceramic braces are better, but still not great. They do appear very close to tooth color; they are essentially transparent and, therefore, less noticeable. However, in order to have the necessary strength, they are larger than the stainless steel brackets and can be a bit more bothersome to the patient's lips and cheeks. They are quite brittle, being made essentially of glass. Therefore, the orthodontist has to be aware to only use very gentle forces with the wires on the brackets in order to move teeth; forgetting this can cause these braces to fracture.

   c.   Invisalign® or other Aligners

This type of treatment consists of a system of clear overlay templates, called aligners, which gradually move crooked teeth into straight teeth.

This system is available to adult patients with certain orthodontic bite problems, but not everyone is a candidate for this type of treatment.

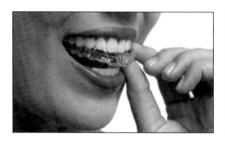 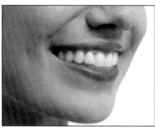

Invisalign uses a series of computer-generated plaster models of the teeth to simulate movement and create proper alignment. The Invisalign Teen System is custom designed specifically for younger patients. This system features a blue-to-clear color-changing dot on the aligners to alert the patient when it is time to go to the next aligner. Again, while not all teens are good candidates for this type of treatment, Invisalign Teen can offer a valuable alternative to conventional braces for most patients.

5. RETAINERS

a. Hawley Retainer

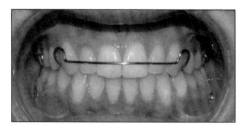 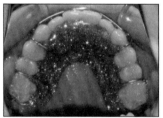

Named for its inventor, Dr. Charles Hawley, the Hawley retainer has stood the test of time and has been around for over ninety years. It consists of an acrylic arch that fits on the roof of the mouth and a wire going around the front of the teeth. The wire can be adjusted to do minor tooth movements. The Hawley retainer's big advantage is that it is very good at holding expansion achieved with The Lauson System. Therefore, we use Hawley retainers at the end of treatment for retention of almost all upper teeth. We sometimes use these for lower teeth as well.

b. Invisible Retainer

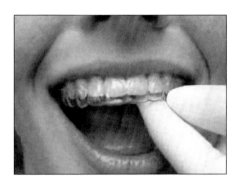

The invisible retainer is excellent for holding teeth alignment, especially the lower front teeth. It is clear and looks like the aligners for Invisalign. It is not as sturdy as a Hawley retainer, but works better to maintain the lower teeth alignment.

c. Fixed Retainers

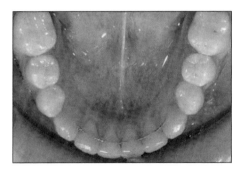

Fixed retainers are bonded to the back sides of the teeth. I rarely use these because a person cannot easily floss between his or her teeth with these retainers in place.

d. Tooth Positioner

A tooth positioner is sometimes used when the teeth need to be settled into a more ideal position. This device is a custom-made, flexible mouthpiece constructed over a precise model of the patient's upper and lower teeth in the exact positions they should ideally occupy. When the patient wears a tooth positioner, he or she bites into the flexible material, forcing the teeth to move into the desired alignment. Tooth positioners are used as an interim appliance between the braces phase and the final retainers in order to achieve a more ideal result than is possible with braces alone. They typically are worn only for a few months immediately after the braces are removed. Patient cooperation is imperative as the teeth are not yet set in the bone structure and their vulnerability to undesirable movement is much higher right after braces are removed. With good patient cooperation, the tooth positioner can help achieve an outstanding result.

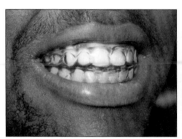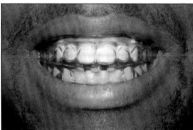

Pertinent Articles and Blogs

1. "ADHD AND SLEEP DISORDERS" FOUND ON WWW.WEBMD.COM

Does your child with ADHD toss and turn all night long? The reason might be a sleep disorder. In a recent study, researchers said that about half the parents in the study said their child with ADHD had difficulty sleeping. Parents reported that their child felt tired on awakening, had nightmares, or had other sleep problems such as sleep apnea or restless legs syndrome. Another study involving children with ADHD found the children had less refreshing sleep, difficulty getting up, and significantly more daytime sleepiness.

Sleep problems and ADHD seem to go hand-in-hand. Let's find out why.

Is snoring related to ADHD?

Large tonsils and adenoids can partially block the airway at night. This can cause snoring, poor sleep quality, and perhaps ADHD.

Because snoring can result in poor sleep, it may lead to attention problems the next day. A study involving five- to seven-year-olds found that snoring is significantly more common among children with mild ADHD, than it is in the general population. In another study, children who snored were almost twice as likely as their peers to have ADHD.

Children who snore perform significantly worse on tests of attention, language abilities, and overall intelligence. Some studies have shown that taking out the tonsils and adenoids may result in better sleep and improved behavior without the need for medications.

What is sleep apnea?

In simplest terms, apnea literally means *without breathing.* The word is used to describe an interruption of airflow of at least ten seconds. While there are three different kinds of apneas, the most common type is obstructive. Obstructive apnea makes up 65% of all apneas.

During obstructive sleep apnea, there is no airflow from the nose and mouth to the lungs. This is because the entrance to the trachea is completely blocked. The cause of the blockage is different structures in the pharynx that have collapsed. During this closure the respiratory muscles continue to make efforts to get air into the lungs.

People with sleep apnea have episodes of breathing cessation. They are aroused then from deep sleep to lighter stages of sleep. But they have these arousals while remaining completely unaware of the apneas or awakenings. These episodes can happen frequently throughout the night.

About 2% of kids in the U.S. have some form of obstructed breathing during sleep. Enlarged tonsils and adenoids are the most common causes of sleep apnea in children. But obesity and chronic allergies can also be a cause. As with adults, children with sleep apnea will be tired during the day. They may have problems concentrating and might have other symptoms related to lack of sleep. For instance, they may display irritability.

How is sleep apnea diagnosed and treated?

Sleep apnea in children is treatable. Yet only your pediatrician or an ear, nose, and throat specialist can determine whether your child's tonsils are enlarged enough to possibly block the airway and cause sleep apnea. Confirmation of sleep apnea should be determined by a polysomnogram. A polysomnogram is a sleep study that's done in a special laboratory. Not every child with enlarged tonsils or with loud snoring has sleep apnea.

Surgery is the treatment of choice for kids with enlarged tonsils and adenoids. Other treatments are available for those with restricted nighttime breathing due to allergies or other causes.

Is restless legs syndrome related to ADHD?

Studies show some correlation between sleep disruption and ADHD and restless legs syndrome (RLS) and ADHD. With restless legs syndrome, there is a creeping, crawling sensation in the legs and sometimes in the arms. This sensation creates an irresistible urge to move. Restless legs syndrome causes sleep disruption and daytime sleepiness.

People with restless legs syndrome and subsequent sleep disruption tell of feeling inattentive, moody, and/or hyperactive—all symptoms of ADHD. Because of this and other findings, some researchers believe that people with restless legs syndrome and a subset of people with ADHD may have a common dysfunction in the neurotransmitter dopamine.

Restless legs syndrome is diagnosed with a polysomnogram or sleep study. Medications can help both restless legs syndrome and ADHD.

How can I help my child with ADHD get the sleep he needs?

It's important to establish a bedtime ritual for children with ADHD. A regular bedtime regimen will help your child relax and get the healthful sleep that's needed. Try these tips:

- **Meet with your doctor and discuss ADHD medications.** Ask your doctor if you can give the morning dose of ADHD medication earlier in the day. Or talk to your doctor about shorter-acting medications. Find the right ADHD medication that lets your child relax at night and get healthy sleep.
- **Be a "no caffeine" family.** Watch for hidden caffeine in your child's diet. Caffeine is one of the few food products that mimic the stress response. When it does, it increases nervousness and causes sleepless nights. Keep caffeinated beverages and foods out of your kitchen.
- **Be consistent.** Have a consistent, daily routine with specific bedtimes, waking times, meals, and family times.
- **Make sure the child's room is sound attenuated.** If your child is bothered by noises while sleeping, try a "white noise" machine. Use one that produces a humming sound or turn the radio to a station that has gone off air. Get earplugs for kids who are extra sensitive to noise.

- **Avoid sleep medications.** If medications are absolutely necessary, talk to your child's doctor about safe and effective treatments.
- **Consider medical problems.** Allergies, asthma, or conditions that cause pain can disrupt sleep. If your child snores loudly and/or pauses in breathing, medical evaluation is necessary. Consult your doctor for help with the possible medical causes of sleep problems.
- **See that your child gets plenty of exercise.** Make sure your child gets daily exercise. But avoid exercising right before bedtime. Studies show that regular exercise helps people sleep more soundly.
- **Give your child a hot bath well before bedtime.** Sleep usually follows the cooling phase of the body's temperature cycle. After your child takes a bath, keep the temperature in your child's bedroom cool to see if you can influence this phase.

2. "PARKINSON'S DISEASE & TMJ: A MYSTERIOUS CONNECTION"

by S. Kent Lauson, DDS, MS and David T. Grove, DDS, MS

Posted on May 23, 2011 by Aurora Orthodontics & TMJ on AOTMJ blog

Strange as it may seem, there is increasing evidence that people diagnosed with Parkinson's disease have the likelihood of having TMJ (jaw joint) dysfunctions and that proper treatment of this disorder by a qualified dentist can help alleviate the symptoms of the disease. At a recent conference sponsored by the Parkinson's Resource Organization & American Academy of Craniofacial Pain, speakers representing various medical disciplines, including dentistry, orthopedic surgery, chiropractic, and neurology relayed remarkable case studies and explanations of how neurologic disorders can be caused by problems with the jaw joint. Although they were quick to point out that this is *not a cure* for Parkinson's disease, the results of a correction of jaw dysfunction in many cases have been astounding, with all typical symptoms of Parkinson's disease being reduced or eliminated. (Those symptoms include a long list going well beyond the hand and body tremors and slow movement or shuffling of feet.) What is particularly exciting is that this type of treatment does not use drugs with all their side effects, but involves the strategic use of a special mouthpiece called a mandibular orthotic to correct the jaw relationship.

When the relationship of the jaw is corrected, many nerves and blood vessels at the back of the jaw joint are no longer being pinched and can be restored to normal function. You see, the area in the back part of the jaw joint accounts for blood vessels that go directly to the brain and nerves that account for a high percentage of neural impulses to the brain. We know that Parkinson's patients have a low amount of dopamine in the brain, a necessary neurotransmitter or an ingredient that allows normal brain function. Incidentally, people with ADHD also are low in dopamine and may be helped by this treatment. This lack of dopamine can be the result of chronic brain stress due to postural misalignment body structures, especially the jaw joints (TMJs) and the bite, since a strong neural and vascular connection to the brain exists in the jaw joints.

Dentists who specialize in this type of treatment are available in most cities of a decent size. The dentists who do this type of treatment can be found through one of these organizations:

1. American Academy of Craniofacial Pain, call 800.322.8651 or online at www.aacf.org

2. International College of Craniomandibular Disorders, call 800.446.1763 or online at www.iccmo.org

For information about Parkinson's Resource Organization, call 877.775.4111 or online at www.parkinsonsresource.org

Or for further information, the authors can be reached at:

Contact information:

Dr. S. Kent Lauson, Aurora Orthodontics & TMJ
24301 E. Orchard Rd., Aurora, CO 80016
303.690.0100
www.aotmj.com

Dr. David T. Grove, Next Generation Education

10408 Mezzanino Court, Las Vegas, NV 89135

702.278.8700

www.nged.org

3. "MEGATRENDS IN ORTHODONTICS"

By S. Kent Lauson, DDS, MS, Orthodontist

Posted on September 1st, 2011 on AOTMJ Blog

Orthodontics has become a commonly anticipated process for many families. However, in my upcoming book, *Straight Talk about Crooked Teeth*, I share my philosophies and treatment procedures that can educate potential patients so that they can make a more informed decision about treatment for their family. The release of this book is timely as the field of orthodontics is in the process of making major changes. Orthodontists are seeing these changes take place, but many are slow to react to them. There are three major trends that are true game changers, as I see them:

MEGATREND #1: INVISALIGN TEEN®

Invisalign as a whole is without question a major game changer and I personally believe that it will radically change the way orthodontics is delivered. It is a treatment whose time has come. Wearing clear plastic aligners twenty-two hours a day to apply a gentle pressure to teeth to straighten them has been a revolution in the field.

Align Technology, the manufacturer of Invisalign, along with key orthodontic providers, introduced Invisalign Teen to the orthodontic/dental community in 2008. They did so with some degree of reservation, presuming that the teens would not be responsible enough to wear their aligners properly and that they would lose their aligners as well. This was based on the established habit patterns of teens wearing braces versus the adult patient. The adult patient was shown to be much more responsible when it came to wearing braces. Because of this it was decided that the teen program should allow a closer monitoring of the progress of the patient. Therefore the program for Invisalign Teen was set up to compensate for this perceived likely cooperation problem by making the aligners with sensing devices built in that could tell the orthodontist that the teen was wearing the aligners as directed. It was also built into the treatment protocol that the loss of a few aligners would not result in extra charges. This would be a comforting factor for the concerned parent.

As it turned out, however, during the last couple years those fears have not been founded in reality. In fact, the cooperation levels of the teens have been found to be as good as their adult counterparts. In addition to that, because of their younger age, their teeth actually responded sooner in their desired movement than the adult teeth did. Interesting!

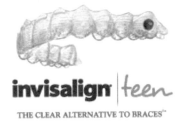

invisalign teen

THE CLEAR ALTERNATIVE TO BRACES™

It seems that the statement *"Braces are for Kids, but Teens prefer Invisalign"* is indeed the answer to the root of the cooperation problem. In studies that put the question of having braces to the teenage boy or girl, it was revealed that 85% of the teenagers would rather not have braces to straighten their teeth at all. In other words, once they become teens, they really want nothing to do with braces and would rather have crooked teeth than tolerate the braces to fix them.

In the past a teen had little choice with an overbearing parent wanting what is best for his or her child saying, "Johnny, you have no choice in the matter. You are going to have braces." This led to many family revolts that occurred even right in the front of the doctor; not a good situation. Orthodontists have long known that the most desirable age to do orthodontic treatment is in the age range of eight to twelve years. Of course, until recently, we have just had the traditional braces to use for all age groups, including teenagers. We as a group always have encouraged parents of children to have the treatment completed by around the child's twelfth birthday.

By then, the twelfth-year molars have come into the patient's mouth and orthodontics can be completed. Of course there are variations of eruption patterns among different individuals, but I think you get the picture. The treatment should be completed by around age twelve so the family unit is left intact. We have long known that the teenager is not as good of a patient as the preteen. Teen psychology has a lot to do with this, but I won't get into that here as there are many books written about the subject.

So now enter **Invisalign Teen**. Over the past couple years that Invisalign Teen has been available, several observations can be made:

1. Invisalign Teen has not only been accepted by the teenage patient, it has been enthusiastically endorsed. Many "Hollywood" teen stars are wearing their aligners and there is quite a buzz about the "invisible" treatment.

2. Orthodontic and dental practices who have accepted this form of treatment are seeing a great deal of growth in their practices. Patients refer other teenagers and seem to be proud of the fact that they have their aligners and nothing is obvious. With braces, teenagers rarely say, "You have to see my orthodontist!" Most teens are already through with treatment, and it is no longer cool.

3. Align Technology as a company is moving forward with this treatment and is providing strong educational support to its doctor providers. This is a trend that isn't going away.

4. Invisalign as a brand name is now the most recognized brand with anything to do with teeth. Patients are asking for it and being referred by Align Technology through its website to the top providers.

5. Invisalign treatment has improved greatly since being introduced in 1999. Every year has seen substantial changes in the technology allowing for advancements in the manufacturing process. Orthodontists and dentists using Invisalign are themselves gaining a great deal of experience and they are successfully treating much more difficult cases than even a couple years ago. I have personally been

surprised at the complexity of the cases that are being successfully resolved without sacrificing the treatment result.

6. In the past, most doctors charged more for Invisalign treatment as they had substantial lab costs associated with the treatment. They reasoned that they would have to pass along the cost to the consumer. However, the trend has been to lower the cost due to less overhead being required as there are fewer patient visits and less time for these visits. No need to change wires or replace loose braces! Lately many of the orthodontists/dentists doing Invisalign and Invisalign Teen are charging the same as treatment with braces. This, when given a choice, certainly will lead the average consumer to choose Invisalign over traditional braces. The consumer, rightly so, perceives the aligner corrections to be a "high tech" type of treatment that may be more costly to produce. However, I predict that there may be a time in the not-too-distant future that the Invisalign and Invisalign Teen treatment may be less costly to the consumer than braces, just like many other high tech items have become less costly over the years.

7. It is important to note that even though Invisalign Teen is making a major move on the scene of orthodontics today, the objectives of The Lauson System, explained in my book, remain intact. All of the principles that I have talked about still need to be the objective of the orthodontist and dentist doing orthodontics. That includes the keys that make it necessary to use FFO prior to Invisalign or braces to achieve the desired results. Invisalign may replace the braces part, but will not replace necessary treatment for the FFO part or more complex corrections, such as for TMJ dysfunction or obstructive sleep apnea. However, as complicated as it may seem, the replacement of the braces part is a very major accomplishment and therefore holds great promise for Invisalign and Invisalign Teen. Stay tuned. For current information on this great technology, see our website at www.AuroraInvisalignDentist.com.

MEGATREND #2: 3D CONE BEAM X-RAY MACHINE

The 3D cone beam x-ray machine is also a true game changer. It is new technology that dentists, oral surgeons, and orthodontists use to view facial structures in 3D. It uses cone beam technology, which reduces the radiation for the patient, to get images that are like seeing through and through the patient's anatomy.

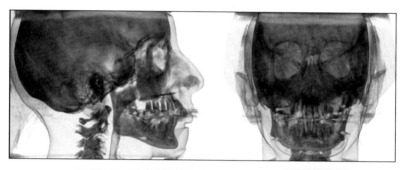

It can show things that were not possible with the older 2D x-ray films. The advantages are significant. It is now the standard of care for many procedures, such as the surgical placement of implants. It allows the surgeon to see all the anatomy, such as nerves, that should be avoided in placement of an implant. It allows the preplanning of those implants to use precision guides for placing multiple implants, even entire mouth implants, in a safe and efficient manner reducing office visits to a minimum. You may have seen ads advertising same-day placement of implanted teeth. This has now become a reality due to cone beam technology.

Although for orthodontic treatment, the use of 3D cone beam imaging has not yet become the standard of care, it may be the standard in the future. Currently, only a tiny percentage of orthodontists have such a machine, but most all have access through x-ray labs in the major cities. Orthodontic uses include the visualization of impacted teeth, especially canine teeth, where their movement can jeopardize adjacent teeth. The 3D image allows the practitioner to visualize how the tooth can be moved to avoid unintended consequences of adverse tooth movements to cause damage to those adjacent teeth. We as orthodontists have always had to rely on the oral surgeon to look directly at the teeth during the actual surgery and then report back to us as to what type of movement is possible.

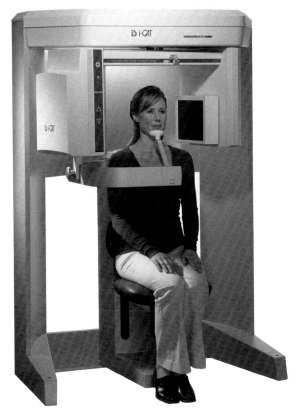

The 3D image eliminates a lot of this guesswork. The orthodontist also can view roots on teeth that have unusual anatomy. As an example, a tooth root may veer off to one direction and present a difficulty in getting an ideal correction in that area. A 3D image can also show extra teeth or aberrations in the bone structure. It shows the thickness of the bone structures that may become important when moving teeth into a precarious area. Another very important area is the great detail it gives of the temporomandibular joint (TMJ). Older 2D topographic x-rays do not do justice when viewing the jaw joints compared to the new 3D views.

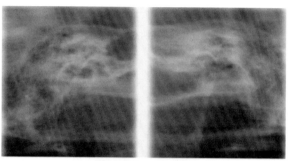

Traditional 2D

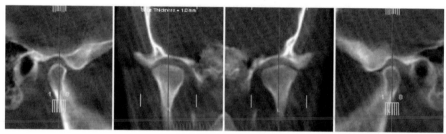

Cone Beam 3D

Another area of great importance is the evaluation of the upper airway in orthodontic patients. The cone beam x-ray, in addition to showing the skeletal anatomy or hard tissue, can also show some of the desired soft tissue anatomy, namely the upper air passageway. This becomes very important in working for the avoidance of obstructive sleep apnea. This is something I believe every dentist doing orthodontics should be aware of and concerned with regarding the future health of his or her patients.

MEGATREND #3: TEMPORARY ANCHORAGE DEVICES (TADs)

In recent years, the use of temporary anchorage devices, or TADs, has become very popular in orthodontics. These are very tiny implants placed by the dentist to help move teeth.

Orthodontists always talk about anchorage. What really is anchorage? Well, to understand the principle of anchorage is to understand why the TADs have become popular. The concept is based on the law of physics that states "for every action there is an equal and opposite reaction." When wanting a tooth (or teeth) to move in a particular direction, the orthodontist has to "anchor" from other teeth to have something to pull or push against. This is a principle the dentist doing orthodontics has to deal with for each patient. Many tooth movements can be planned to pit one tooth or set of teeth against the other to create a positive change for both. This includes an understanding of the "law of unintended consequences." There can be adverse tooth movements as well, which are undesirable. This is where TADs come in.

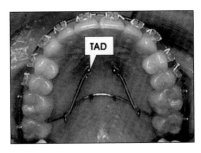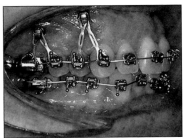

TADs can be used to anchor on a stable part of the bone structure. Think of them as mini-implants, because that is exactly what they are. They are strategically placed in the bone by gently screwing them in. They are very tiny so don't create a lot of discomfort. Implants essentially can't be moved with orthodontic forces, so the mini-implants won't move either. Therefore, teeth can be moved by pulling on these TADs and the TADs remain in the same place. Pretty cool, huh? Once the teeth have moved and the TAD is no longer needed, the TAD is removed by gently unscrewing it and the area is allowed to heal. That is why they are called temporary. The desired correction has been achieved without the need for surgery or extraction of permanent teeth. This is a good thing. TADs are around to stay and are the third megatrend in orthodontics today. Even though TADs can be a great tool for orthodontics, the importance of The Lauson System and the Nine Keys to Lower Facial Harmony, as explained in my book, are not to be ignored.

4. "PROTANDIM, A BREAKTHROUGH ANTI-AGING AND HEALTH PRODUCT"

Protandim is arguably the biggest breakthrough of any supplement in the last century.

Founded in science; developed with forty years of research; confirmed by nine independent, peer-review studies at leading universities; featured on ABC, NBC, PBS, and in the *Wall Street Journal*; described in CNN Chief Medical Correspondent Dr. Sanjay Gupta's book *Chasing Life*; and available exclusively through LifeVantage, Protandim is specially formulated to fight aging at the source, the body's own cells.

Protandim has been scientifically proven to reduce oxidative stress, which is caused by the body's overproduction of free radicals by an average of forty percent in thirty days in anyone who takes the product. This is done by delivering a biochemical wake-up call to each of the several trillion cells in a person's body to increases production of protective genes called survival genes. It also decreases production of the genes that can cause inflammation and scar tissue formation. Almost all degenerative diseases, including heart disease and cancer, result from inflammation, a direct result of oxidative stress caused by the attack of free radicals, which occur in every cell in our body. Protandim causes the body to drastically reduce inflammation and free-radical damage, boosting the immune system to help protect against disease, with the potential of adding years of healthy living to one's life.

Montel Williams, well known for having an MS condition in the past and an advocate for healthy living, is a strong proponent of taking his daily Protandim. He has made public his endorsement: "This product fits so perfectly with what I am trying to do to make people's lives better. Once people get information about this product, it is going to do so much good on so many levels." Donny Osmond also publically endorses Protandim and states: "I love Protandim, I take it every day! I have personally experienced the health-promoting benefits of Protandim and feel compelled to share it."

Why is this information talked about in our orthodontic office? The reduction of inflammation is very important in the dental field since it plays such a dominant role in virtually all dental related diseases, including the critical area of periodontal disease, which has now been linked to heart disease. At Aurora Orthodontics & TMJ, we recommend Protandim because we know that, in addition to the other great health benefits, reducing inflammation in the gums during orthodontic treatment can speed up orthodontics and provide a more comfortable process for the patient. Also, virtually all types of pain, including TMJ and headache pain, can be reduced by taking Protandim.

A valuable link to investigate Protandim is www.abcliveit.com.

You also can read the nine peer-reviewed papers at www.pubmed.gov (just type in "Protandim" or what it addresses, "oxidative stress," with some 87,825 papers on this subject).

For ordering or to become a distributor of Protandim, visit www.Mylifevantage.com/auroraorthodontics.

For Dental and Medical Professionals

1. "A NEW GOLD STANDARD FOR ORTHODONTIC EVALUATIONS"

by S. Kent Lauson, DDS, MS, Aurora, Colorado

During my thirty-five years in the private practice of orthodontics, I have many times asked myself the question, "Are we as doctors in the field of dentistry (and specifically within orthodontics) doing all we can to create the best result possible?" When I talk about "the best result possible," I am not limiting my assessment to just teeth and jaw joints. Let's think outside the box for a minute. Because the teeth are connected (either directly or indirectly) to many other structures in the head and neck, it could be that what we do with the teeth can affect these other areas. It is my understanding that we do indeed affect these other areas in a very profound way every day in our orthodontic practices. Since this is the case, then how can we affect these other areas in a positive way, and how can we avoid any unwarranted side effects from our treatment? Always remember the Hippocratic Oath, which tells us to do no harm to our patients. I know that a thorough understanding of the effects of what we do can allow us to provide care far beyond the pleasing aesthetic results of straight teeth that we are so famous for. To treat patients is our right and privilege by the license that we hold, and I believe it is our obligation to provide the finest treatment we are capable of as well.

Because a thorough understanding of any problem (proper diagnosis) is needed before finding a way to fix it (proper treatment plan), the evaluation of the patient becomes critical. Therefore, I have put together a protocol that I use every day when evaluating a new patient. This has evolved over the past thirty-plus years into essentially the following:

1. Standard Orthodontic Evaluation

    a. Angle classification (molar or cuspid, if different)

    b. Overbite and overjet

    c. Dental crowding and spacing

    d. Arch form assessment (ideal or narrow width, etc.)

    e. Dental protrusion or retrusion

    f. Skeletal protrusion or retrusion

    g. Relationship of upper jaw to lower jaw

    h. Crossbite

    i. Dental wear patterns

    j. Missing, extra, or abnormal tooth development

    k. Periodontal health assessment

    l. Aesthetic vertical (This is a measurement I use of millimeters of gingival tissue showing with the patient smiling fully in laughter mode.)

    m. Recognition of any adverse habits such as thumb or finger sucking, poor tongue posture, or mouth breathing

    n. Photos (eight total) and panoramic x-ray used for further study

2. TMJ Assessment

    a. Patient history to include headaches, pain, or dysfunction around the head and neck areas (We track over sixty different symptoms with our TMJ patients.)

    b. Measurement of range of motion (ROM) (Opening normal is 45–55mm and side normals are 10–12mm. These movements should be smooth [absence of dyskensia].)

    c. Assessment of joint noise during ROM movements with palpation and/or stethoscope (I have used more advanced techniques such as Doppler, but do not feel these are necessary.)

    d. Bilateral muscle palpations to include the following:

        i. Anterior and posterior temporalis

        ii. Posterior cervical muscles at nuchal line

        iii. Sternocleidomastoid (SCM)

        iv. Scalenes

        v. Anterior digastrics

        vi. Trapezius

        vii. TMJ palpation, both internal and lateral

        viii. Advanced muscle assessments with full electromyography (EMG) studies (I have used these but do not feel they are necessary and are an unnecessary expense to the patient.)

    e. Radiographic evaluation to the TMJs (Over the years, I have successfully used tomograms for this assessment; however, recent developments of cone beam computerized tomography (CBCT) have prompted me to currently have an i-Cat machine to give an even better TMJ assessment.)

3. Upper Airway Assessment (Note the presence of nasopharyngeal obstruction, which leads to a mouth-breathing habit.)

    a. Patient history of snoring, obstructive sleep apnea, or mouth breathing

    b. Visual assessment of patient to include:

        i. Lip posture (open or closed)

        ii. Dryness of lips, tongue (coating)

        iii. Dull, apathetic look

    c. Evaluation of tonsils (seen visually at the back of the throat) and adenoids (seen on Ceph)

    d. Previously noted upper arch form (It has a great deal to do with upper airway competence in that the palatal bone at the roof of the mouth is also the floor of the nasal air passageway.)

    e. Notation of allergic shiners, if present (Allergic rhinitis can be a cause of upper-airway obstruction.)

    f. Radiographic evaluation of airway patency with CBCT (It can be very helpful, especially when treating patients with obstructive sleep apnea.)

4. Head Postural Observation (A mouth-breathing habit always results in a forward head posture. It is almost always present with a TMJ dysfunction or obstructive sleep apnea patient as well. Chiropractors will tell you that a forward head posture is very damaging to a person's neck and back health and is one of the hardest things to correct. Once they know that orthodontics can help by changing occlusal patterns, they are glad to refer patients to us. Radiologic evaluation of the neck with a cephalometric or cone beam x-ray machine can help to evaluate the health of the cervical spine, including looking for normal lordosis, which is lost with chronic forward head posture.)

THE VALUE OF "A NEW GOLD STANDARD FOR ORTHODONTIC EVALUATIONS"

About twenty-five years ago I set myself on a path to discover what was missing from my orthodontic education and why I felt inadequate when I would hear the next guru speak. They all seemed somewhat convincing, but many were in conflict. Their ideologies would clash and some of these intellectual titans would revel in putting down another titan who somehow missed a minute point in a presentation.

I spent the next five years studying all types of philosophies and always tried to ask myself, "Does this make sense?" To be sure, I learned a great deal from these leaders, but by the time I had surpassed over 2,500 hours and five years of additional continuing education, I felt that I knew more than most of the speakers out there, at least in terms of what *I* felt was important. I still wasn't confident enough or motivated enough to place my philosophies out there for all to see. I needed more time and more clinical experience.

That was then. This is now, over twenty-five years later. During the senior years of my practice life I have decided to disseminate the information that, as I see it, can change and expand the role of orthodontics in the world of medicine. Our patients need our help more than we can imagine. Although dentists, in general, have much work to do before we can become the great healers we all have the potential to be, the rewards are definitely worth the effort.

A quote from one of my recent patients speaks to the life-changing results in our power to bestow: "It was absolutely amazing. Whenever I had the mouthpiece in, my symptoms would disappear. I could not believe that Dr. Lauson addressed the problem in one hour—something that five years of doctors, tests, x-rays, MRIs, chiropractors, psychologists, and a Mayo Clinic visit could not do."

This is not an isolated happening. I have had countless patients share with me that our work has changed their lives for the better. In our office, we are constantly rewarded with glowing tributes to the beautiful, new smile that has given a son or daughter renewed confidence. Although this is gratifying, naturally, and we all are truly blessed to be able to do orthodontics, I am talking about the much greater healing role that we can play in helping our fellow man. It all begins with a comprehensive exam and a treatment plan that gives us the roadmap to achieve a patient's optimal result.

2. DR. LAUSON'S REVIEW OF BOOK: *EPIGENETIC ORTHODONTICS IN ADULTS*

This breakthrough book, *Epigenetic Orthodontics in Adults,* has recently been published for the orthodontic profession. It puts into scientific terms the rationale behind the efficacy of FFO, which is the cornerstone of my treatment philosophy. This text provides the scientific basis for much of the treatment shown in this book.

The authors give a compelling argument for the new theory of "Spatial Matrix Hypothesis," which relies on Moss' Functional Matrix hypothesis as a starting point. They talk about the fact that a majority of adults have an underdevelopment of the midface area of the skull due to "epigenetic" (gene-environmental) factors, resulting in smaller-than-ideal dental arch formations and subsequent crowding of teeth and overbites. They further explain: *"Growth mechanisms, and not growth outcome, are defined by the human genome."* Environmental factors also can play a huge role. Dominant environmental factors can be as diverse as the force and frequency of mastication or a habitual mouth-breathing habit, which leads to the developmental problems discussed previously in this book in Key #2: Unobstructed Nasal Breathing.

The authors state: *"Aside from the cosmetic detractions, other conditions of co-morbidity may exist in these cases (of midface underdevelopment), such as Temporomandibular Dysfunction, headaches, snoring, sleep disordered breathing, and frank Obstructive Sleep Apnea (OSA), which results in an expected decrease in longevity associated with hypertension, cardiac disease, diabetes, and cerebro-vascular incidents (strokes), etc. These serious, life-threatening consequences make the diagnosis of facial underdevelopment mandatory for the modern dental professional. Thus, as snoring, upper airway resistance syndrome, sleep disordered breathing, and OSA are associated with malocclusions (and constricted maxillas), they should also be viewed as indicators of decreased longevity, and efforts should be made to address the causative conditions."*

The authors further state: *"Patients with underdeveloped faces can have a narrow, high-vaulted hard palate, whereas patients with good (ideal) facial development have wide arches."* They also point out that constricted and obstructed nasal passageways can be the result of narrow maxillary arches, and that *"obstruction of the pharyngeal airway space can be fatal in the adult and child alike. Sudden Infant Death Syndrome (SIDS) may be associated with under-development of the pharyngeal airway. While further research is required on SIDS, Nocturnal Enuresis (bed wetting) is a more common condition in younger children, and may be precipitated by nighttime oxygen deprivation. The decreased oxygen saturation may fall beyond a threshold, which results in an acute hypoxic episode associated with 'hypoxic stress,' which leads to a fight or flight reaction with loss of bladder tone due to vasopressin release."* Also, *". . . these children may demonstrate nighttime snoring as they grow older and develop obstructive sleep apnea as older adults."*

"Underdeveloped faces may indicate a collapse or constriction of the upper pharyngeal airway space." Stated later: *"Obstruction of the upper airway space can be due to enlarged tonsils"* or adenoids. *"In the past tonsillectomy was carried out routinely; while it remains as an elective treatment, it is less commonly performed these days even though it may be of immense value in preventing the onset of chronic mouth breathing."* Also, *". . . patients adopt peculiar cervical curvatures (loss of Cervical Lordosis with forward head posture) in order to preserve the upper airway space."* The book talks about the *". . . significance of sutures during craniofacial development,"* and how properly placed light tension at the sutures creates *". . . a physiologic response which ultimately leads to bone deposition at those sites."* Also, *". . . recent research suggests that these sutures persist throughout adult life and provide a developmental mechanism for continued maxillofacial morphogenesis via mechano-transduction."*

Perhaps the most significant finding reported in the book is that slow palatal expansion (only about one activation of ¼ millimeter per week) is the most physiologic and ideal stimulation for midface/palatal expansion.

I have found that through the use of craniosacral midpalatal suture release techniques practiced daily by the patient, a physiologic activation of twice a week can be done very successfully. This slow activation stimulates the differentiation of stem cells located within the sutures to form osteoblasts, leading to true bone formation. Conversely, the prevailing method used today in orthodontics, that of rapid palatal expansion (RPE), has substantial side effects and unintended consequences. Side effects reported in the book include "tearing of the osteogenic periosteum at the midpalatal suture, accompanied by mild hemorrhage and pain." The healing may result in collagenous tissue and scar formation. This scar tissue can contract as the child grows older and can account, in part, for the relapse encountered many times in the use of an RPE protocol.

The authors state: *"Perhaps the greatest benefit of expansion is simply unlocking the cranial keys to achieve optimum development, and perhaps the orthodontist's highest function may be to recapture space in all the right areas to allow the latent genes to be reactivated. The human genome is millions of years old, while the compromised phenotype of mid-facial underdevelopment is a feature of the last few hundred years of human development."* The authors also recommend that dental professionals *". . . visualize each person as a potentially perfect being in form and function and ask 'why not?' to get to the cause of the problem."*

The conclusions listed at the end of the book are as follows:

1. Osteogenetic-orthodontics does not rely upon surgery, drugs, or injections.

2. Osteogenetic-orthodontics involves foundational correction with or without a simultaneous functional correction.

3. Sutural homeostasis corrects malocclusions in adults by remodeling the maxilla and mandible, in accord with the Spatial Matrix hypothesis.

4. Enhancement of craniofacial homeostasis in adults does not mandate extractions or interproximal reduction.

5. Circum-maxillary sutural remodeling can produce natural improvements in the facial features of passively growing adults, commensurate with a nonsurgical facelift to enhance facial aesthetics.

6. Osteogenetic-orthodontics is associated with physiologic functional improvements at the TMJ.

7. Osteogenetic-orthodontics is associated with functional improvements in the upper airway.

8. Osteogenetic-orthodontics is noninvasive and allows the body to naturally gain an enhanced level of craniofacial homeostasis, in accord with physiologic principles.

Epigenetic Orthodontics in Adults is a very important book for any practitioner in the field of orthodontics. It opens the door to understanding the possibilities in the treatment we can give our patients. In conjunction with this book, *Straight Talk about Crooked Teeth*, it can transform how orthodontics is performed today and give our patients a real advantage in living a much more healthy and longer life.

Epigenetic Orthodontics in Adults by Professor G. David Singh and Dr. James A. Krumholtz is available from:

> Smile Foundation
> Appliance Therapy Group
> 9139 Lurline Avenue
> Chatsworth, CA 91311
> 800.423.3270
> www.SMILEFoundation.com

3. "IN SEARCH OF IMPROVED SKELETAL TRANSVERSE DIAGNOSIS"

by Dr. John L. Hayes, Orthodontist
(Review by Dr. S. Kent Lauson, Orthodontist)

Part One: In his two-part article, Dr. Hayes emphasizes that there is no accepted uniform standard in evaluating the transverse dimension in the maxillary dental arch and skeletal bone structure. Many methods have been used, but none have come forward to be the "gold standard." He feels that cone beam CT scans have the potential to become this standard. The shortcomings of present methods include the buccal tipping of maxillary posterior teeth in many cases when a maxillary deficiency exists. Lower posterior teeth will then tend to tip lingually. This compensates for the narrow upper jaw and prevents the formation of a posterior crossbite. A new standard of measuring these relationships is needed.

Part Two: This part of the article suggests using a new method of measuring the transverse dimension of the upper jaw by using dental study casts to determine the center of the alveolar crest (CAC) at the first molar area measured to the CAC on the opposite side. From the author's previous studies of old and prehistoric skulls (derived from museums around the world), the conclusion was that the dental occlusions with these skulls were ideal and their maxillas possessed an ideal U-shape without crowding of the dentition. No V-shaped narrow maxillas were found among this prehistoric group of skulls. The CACs of the old maxillas were nearly uniformly 5mm wider than the CACs of the mandibles. Using this criterion (+5mm for maxillary CAC compared to mandibular CAC) for his study, the author examined 114 pretreatment patients. One hundred and eight of the 114 consecutive pretreatment patients in the study were shown to be maxillary skeletal transverse deficient. Dr. Hayes' conclusion was that maxillary skeletal transverse deficiency may be more prevalent than previously thought. The severity of the deficiency varied, with expansion needed to achieve an ideal varying from 5mm to as much as 17mm.

Comments: This is a very good study that points out the prevalence of maxillary deficiency in today's society. Although the author's 114 pretreatment patients perhaps fairly represent the subset of people seeking orthodontic treatment, it cannot be assumed that this high incidence of maxillary deficiency (around 95%) would exist throughout the population in general. I am sure that the percentage in the general population would be much lower. However, it is likely that dental crowding and overbites, the two main reasons for which a patient seeks orthodontic treatment, are likely caused by an underdeveloped maxilla. This to me seems very reasonable and a probable explanation of why Dr. Hayes had such a high rate of maxillary deficiency in his study. In other words, people seeking orthodontic treatment likely have a very high incidence (95% in Dr. Hayes' study) of maxillary transverse deficiency. It seems then logical that this maxillary deficiency should be corrected prior to alignment of the teeth. This is where dentofacial orthopedics should come in and is in direct alignment with the recommendations of this book. I have previously stated that almost all patients seeking treatment from an orthodontist should have a dentofacial orthopedic phase prior to the teeth-straightening phase. We as orthodontists must always ask the question, "How did the teeth end up this way?" Many times the cause is that of an underdeveloped maxilla or other orthopedic misalignment. Therefore, straightening the skeletal alignment prior to straightening of the teeth is critical.

It is noteworthy that the article also states that long-term stability with the use of RPEs to correct these maxillary deficiencies was not very successful. Dr. Hayes writes: "The dental relapse phenomenon is not new information. In some cases the relapse was 30% of that measured by turn-buckle (a modified Haas design); in other cases it was more than 50%. Measurements were taken at least 6 weeks post-RPE removal compared to measurements of the patient's RPE turnbuckle expansion." In my opinion, this is compelling evidence of the power of slow palatal expansion (SPE) rather than RPE.

For a complete copy of the printed magazine and article listed, please contact:

> Orthodontic Practice US
> 15720 N. Greenway Hayden Loop #9
> Scottsdale, AZ 85260
> Telephone 866.579.9496
> Ask for: Volume 1, Numbers 3 and 4
> Or contact Dr. Hayes directly at: jhayesortho@comcast.net

4. "THE OCCLUSAL-TMJ-CERVICAL CONNECTION"

by S. Kent Lauson, DDS, MS

Presented at the Annual Meeting of the American Association of Orthodontists – May 1990, Washington, D.C.

also

Presented at the Sixth Annual International Symposium on Clinical Management of Head, Neck, Facial Pain and TMJ Disorders – August 1990, Philadelphia, PA

Those of us involved in treating temporomandibular and myofacial pain dysfunctions are very aware that neckaches and backaches are a common complaint among these patients. The purpose of this presentation is to show how occlusion can play a major role in TMD/MPD and can play a strong role in cervical (neck) dysfunction.

There are many etiologic factors that can produce craniomandibular dysfunctions. However, with the exception of trauma, most come as a result of occlusion. For occlusion itself to cause TMD/MPD, it must be incompatible with proper unrestrained presence of retrusive occlusal contacts. A retrusive contact is any contact that lessens or stops when the mandible is closed in a more retruded position. Retrusive contacts can slow the growth of the mandible (for those still growing) and cause posterior displacement of the condyles.

It is well known that people with deep overbites are predisposed to TMD. Deep overbites can be due to lack of posterior vertical development and/or super eruption of anteriors, causing premature anterior contacts on closure. If lack of vertical and anterior super eruption are both present, the person will likely have the lower bicuspids at a lower level than the cuspids (due to lack of posterior vertical development) and more than normal attrition on all anteriors, cuspid to cuspid. When this is present, comprehensive neuromuscular orthodontics is highly indicated.

Class II malocclusions, even without deep overbites, also predispose a person to TMD. This is because most Class IIs have some constriction in the maxilla and, therefore, a constriction in the maxillary teeth and the creation of buccal retrusive contacts. A neuromuscular message is sent to the brain by the proprioceptive nerve endings in the periodontal ligaments of the teeth. The retrusion occurs through hyperactivity of mandibular retruders (suprahyoids and posterior temporalis). Bruxing and clenching (hyperactivity of masseters, pterygoids, and temporalis) can occur as the grinding mechanism attempts to relieve premature or retrusive contacts. This is the body's response when the fit of the teeth does not match with proper unrestrained function of the temporomandibular joints. This hyperactivity of the masticatory muscle can be accessed by palpating these muscles for tenderness and size or, more accurately, by evaluating them through electromyography (EMG).

Hyperactivity can lead to excess attrition, and, moreover, to closure and subsequent shortening of masticatory muscles. The muscles can become painful due to lactic acid building up from overuse. The TMJ disc can become displaced. The displacement is due to the following factors, either singly or in combination: 1) retrusive positioning of mandible resulting in posterior displacement of the condyles; 2) masticatory muscles' overactivity and shortening causing superior position of the condyles and TMJ compression; 3) hyperactivity of superior head of the lateral pterygoids. This important muscle inserts on and pulls the disc anterior and medial to cause anterior-medial displacement of the disc. The posterior and/or superior position of the condyles can result in compression and mechanical entrapment of the critical neurovascular bundle within the retrodiscal tissue.

Because branches of the fifth and seventh cranial nerves and key arteries pass through this area, significant pain and dysfunction can occur, including but not limited to the following symptoms:

1. Headaches, facial pain, difficulty chewing
2. Ears – ringing, fullness, pain, hearing loss
3. Eyes – blurring, pain, light sensitivity, watering

The TMJ internal derangement eventually leads to osteoarthritic, cartilaginous, and soft tissue changes within the TMJ.

While all the previously described changes within the teeth, masticatory muscles, and TMJ have been occurring, another phenomenon is also taking place. In order to have less straining on the mandibular retruder muscles (anterior digastrics, posterior temporalis), the head accommodates by moving forward of normal ideal posture. This lessens the amount of pull necessary to retrude the mandible.

The occlusal reason for the forward head posture phenomenon can be demonstrated as follows:

1. Stand or sit upright with your head rotated back as far as comfortably possible. Let your lower jaw hang loose, unrestrained, and gently tap your teeth together. Remember where the teeth touch.

2. Now, rotate your head down toward your chest as far as comfortably possible. (Position head as if trying to make a double chin.) With your lower jaw hanging loose and unrestrained, tap your teeth together.

If your teeth fit comfortably in the first position, it is a good bet you have a forward head posture with neckaches, headaches, and backaches likely experienced. During the day, your teeth have to close together many times (reportedly up to 2,000 times a day, just during swallowing). Because you can't go walking around with your head tilted backward so your teeth fit together correctly, you instead compensate by bringing your head forward, which is the same basic neuromuscular relationship of the lower jaw to cranium.

This forward head postural compensation places a heavy strain on the posterior cervical and upper trapezius muscles. This can lead to head, neck, and back aches. Other symptoms can occur, such as numbing of fingers and hands from muscle entrapment (scalene) of the brachial plexus. The constant muscular straining and forward head posturing can also lead to loss of the normal lordotic curvature of the cervical spine. Normal movements of the head and neck are now somewhat restricted. Further progression of this cervical dysfunction can lead to kyphosis (reverse curvature), subluxations of cervical vertebrae, and osteoarthritic degeneration.

APPLICATION OF PRINCIPLES

Postural observations should be made on all patients, especially those where changes in occlusion are contemplated, i.e., orthodontics and prosthodontics. Cervical spine x-rays (cephalometric x-rays showing cervical vertebrae) can be extremely valuable in determining occlusal positions that will help and never cause harm to our patients. When patients undergo restorative, orthodontic, or TMJ treatment, postural evaluations should always be made. Consideration should be given to the questions: Are present occlusal relationships helping or hurting this person's head posture? What can be done to improve or maintain the dynamic relationship of the teeth, lower jaw (and TMJ), and neck? Treatment should include the following:

1. Understand the relationship of occlusion, TMJ, and posture.

2. Always move treatment in the direction of better balance within the stomatognothic/cervical system. Do not equilibrate to lessen vertical dimension on vertically over-closed patients!

3. When working with dysfunctional patients or changing occlusion, do temporary reversible procedures such as orthotics, temporary crowns, and bridges of functional orthopedics.

4. When creating your temporary (or permanent) occlusion, always situate patient upright (not lying down in dental chair) in as correct a posture possible. I place my patients in an exaggeratedly good posture when testing and developing temporary occlusion. This will allow them to move as fast as possible toward better posture to help eliminate neck and back problems.

5. Use sophisticated scientific instrumentation such as computerized electromyography and computerized mandibular tracking to develop and document occlusal relationships.

6. Always have muscles relaxed as much as possible prior to establishing temporary occlusion. The myomonitor (TENS) is quite effective in relaxing muscles (reduce EMG readings to normal) and in allowing them to achieve normal resting length.

Author's note: Although this article was first presented over twenty years ago, I have found the essential principles remain unchanged. However, a thorough understanding of these principles will allow the practitioner to use practiced shortcuts in most cases. Orthodontists are advised to establish a practical approach that takes these principles into consideration, so as not to "run up" the cost for the patient (or the doctor).

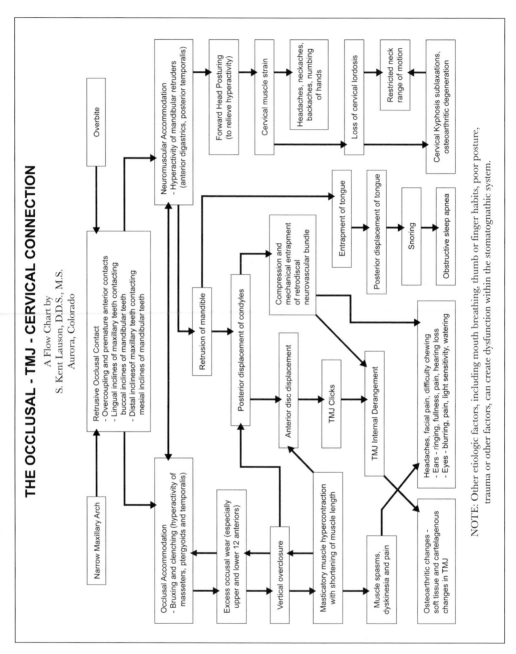

This chart is available for purchase in a larger (11"x17") format suitable for display at www.StraightTalkaboutCrookedTeeth.org.

5. EXCERPT FROM *ORTHODONTICS FOR THE TMJ/TMD PATIENT*

The following is an excerpt from a book titled *Orthodontics for the TMJ/TMD Patient* by Duane Grummons, DDS, MSD, orthodontist. As the name suggests, this book, published in 1994, was written for the orthodontist and discusses the relationship between dysfunction in the TMJ and orthodontics. Chapter 5 of the book, entitled "Abnormal Muscle Forces and Unstable Occlusion: Facial Pain and Orthodontic Solutions," written by Brendan C. Stack, DDS, MS, explains the relationship between the muscles in the head and neck and alignment of the teeth. On pages 107 and 108, Dr. Stack explains:

"Orthodontists are in a unique position to: diagnose these structural joint malalignments; correct them to normal physiologic function, if possible; and then subsequently rearrange the dental occlusion to support and stabilize these restored healthy joints. Orthodontic treatment should then result in a rearranged occlusion that no longer has abnormal muscle forces acting on it since the muscles surrounding the temporomandibular joints are usually at their resting lengths except when functioning. The orthodontically rearranged occlusion would support and harmoniously function with optimally functioning temporomandibular joints in each specific patient. The only other alternative to this concept is to have the occlusion function with abnormal pathological temporomandibular joints or to joints whose status is unknown. A Class I dental occlusion is a desirable and achievable goal. When an ideal, non-orthodontic Class I dentition is observed, the clinician is frequently misled into thinking that the patient's stomatognathic system in general, and his occlusion and temporomandibular joint in particular, are essentially normal. This is not necessarily true.

It has been the author's experience that many Class I occlusions have compensations with unilateral or bilateral chronically displaced disks or "pre-clicking" joints in which both the condyle and the disc are in their normal relationship to each other, but are not in their normal relationship to the posterior slope of the eminence. They are posteriorized within the joint away from the posterior slope of the eminence and constitute what has previously been called "pseudo" Class III patients. These are the Class I occlusions presenting with headache and facial pain, either acute, sub acute, or chronic. Since the "pre-clicking" joint exhibits no recurrent disc dislocation and therefore no audible sounds (clicking) on function, and since there is no non-recurrent disc dislocation (locking) nor impaired range of motion, yet moderate to severe pain is usually present, these conditions have been dismissed and mislabeled as Myofascial Pain Dysfunction (MPD). It is the author's contention that in the absence of overt muscular trauma, Myofascial Pain Dysfunction does not exist as an entity in itself. It exists as a consequence of an intracapsular, special alteration of joint structure in the absence of a specific disc derangement. Both the condyle and its disc become posteriorized within the Glenoid Fossa, causing the masticatory muscles that originate above and around the joint and insert into the periosteum of the mandible below the joint to now have an altered angulation from origin to insertion because the mandible itself is posteriorized. It is a third variation of internal derangement causing subsequent muscle involvement. One's primary efforts should not be in symptomatic treatment of the involved muscles, but in restoring normal spacial positions of the condyle and disc within the fossa.

As orthodontists, we err in accepting a Class I malocclusion as one that is stomatognathically non-pathologic, has an optimal maxillomandibular relationship, and has no abnormal muscle forces associated with it. We routinely do not inquire about sub acute or chronic symptomology nor do we evaluate impaired temporomandibular function. Not recognizing that a Class I malocclusion may have an abnormal maxillomandibular relationship and associated abnormal muscle forces acting on it (the reason it is a malocclusion), the orthodontist proceeds to straighten the malaligned occlusion to existing conditions and preconceived objectives taught in graduate training. He produces a new dental occlusion with the same maxillomandibular malrelationship and abnormal muscle forces present and active. Predictable relapse within 2-5 years after retention is usual and should be expected."

6. AOTMJ SYMPTOMS RATING SHEET

The chart is the list of symptoms I have compiled in order to follow progress when treating patients for TMJ dysfunction. This gives a comprehensive understanding of how the jaw dysfunction is affecting them on an individual basis. Each time they are in the office, they rate their relevant symptoms so that their rate of healing can be accurately tracked. The eventual goal for the totals calculated on each day's entry is to be over a 90% reduction for a period of four to six months before proceeding to the next phase to complete their treatment with FFO/orthodontics.

(See chart next page.)

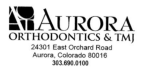

ORTHODONTICS & TMJ
24301 East Orchard Road
Aurora, Colorado 80016
303.690.0100

SYMPTOMS RATING

Patient Name: _____   Date: _____

Please identify those symptoms below that recently pertain to you by rating them according to the following scale:

4=very severe   3=severe   2=moderate   1=mild   0=nonexistent

SYMPTOM   RATING

Headaches	_____	Difficulty closing mouth	_____
Facial pain	_____	Opening deviation of jaw to side	_____
Jaw pain	_____	Popping/Clicking of jaw joint	_____
Jaw joint pain	_____	Grating of jaw joint	_____
Neckaches	_____	Locking of jaw joint	_____
Upper backaches	_____	Ear pain	_____
Lower backaches	_____	Hearing loss	_____
Scoliosis	_____	Ringing in ears	_____
Dizziness/Lightheadedness	_____	Noise sensitivity	_____
Loss of concentration	_____	Fullness in ears/sinuses	_____
Low self-esteem	_____	Pain while eating	_____
Fatigue	_____	Clenching of teeth	_____
Depression	_____	Teeth sensitive to hot/cold	_____
Forgetfulness	_____	Teeth sensitive to chewing	_____
Anxiety/panic attacks	_____	Numbness	_____
Loss of sleep	_____	Allergy problems	_____
Excessive dreaming/nightmares	_____	Mouth breathing habit	_____
Eye pain	_____	Sinus problems	_____
Pain behind the eyes	_____	Mitral valve prolapse	_____
Visual disturbances	_____	Irregular heart beats	_____
Twitching of eyelids	_____	Nausea or upset stomach	_____
Light sensitivity	_____	Neurologic disorders	_____
Post nasal drainage	_____	Type:_____.	
Difficulty swallowing	_____	Other: _____	_____
Chronic sore throat	_____	Other: _____	_____
Difficulty opening mouth	_____	Other: _____	_____
		Total: _____	_____

7. NASOPHARYNGEAL OBSTRUCTION CHART

The following flow chart on nasopharyngeal obstruction (NPO) was created in 1990, primarily for patient education, to emphasize the great importance of having proper nasal breathing. Most people, doctors included, are not aware of the many ramifications of an obstructive nasal passageway. As time has gone on, the verification of the preventable problem of nasopharyngeal obstruction seems today even more relevant as more recent studies have shown the connection to many childhood ills whose association was previously unknown. Those new additions to my chart include ADHD and SIDS.

(See flow chart next page.)

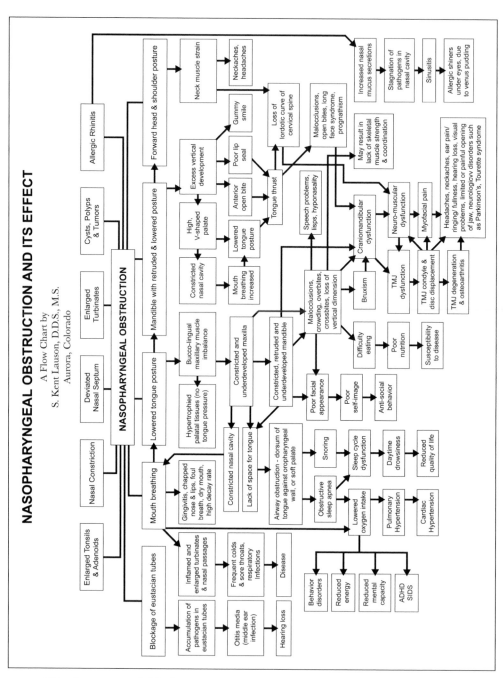

NASOPHARYNGEAL OBSTRUCTION AND ITS EFFECT

A Flow Chart by
S. Kent Lauson, D.D.S., M.S.
Aurora, Colorado

This chart is available for purchase in a larger (11"x17") format suitable for display at www.StraightTalkaboutCrookedTeeth.org.

Glossary

3D cone beam x-ray machine—New technology that dentists, oral surgeons, and orthodontists use to view facial structures in 3D. It uses cone beam technology (reducing radiation for the patient) to get images like seeing through the patient's anatomy.

ADD and **ADHD**—attention deficit (hyperactivity) disorder—A condition occurring mainly in children, it is characterized by the coexistence of the inability to concentrate and impulsive or inappropriate behavior.

CAC–center of the alveolar crest—The middle point where the center of a tooth fits into its bone socket.

CBCT–cone beam computed tomography—The technology behind the 3D cone beam x-ray machine, similar to medical CT scanning but with a small fraction of the radiation.

cervical lordosis—The normal curvature in the cervical (neck) region of the spine.

CMS–computerized mandibular scan—A computer tracking device that records, in three dimensions, the delicate functional movements of the jaw with great accuracy. It is used to create a myocentric orthotic to correct a dysfunction of the jaw.

condyle—The round end of the lower jaw, which fits into the area of the skull that is part of the temporomandibular joint (TMJ).

craniosacral therapy—The specialty of medicine related to normalizing the craniosacral system in the body by using gentle manipulations of the bones of the skull. This system is contained within the dural matter of the spine and brain and contains cerebral spinal fluid.

crepitus—A medical term used to describe the crackling or grating sounds that occur during movement of a joint. This is a common symptom of an advanced TMJ dysfunction caused by bone-on-bone contact.

crossbite—An abnormal relationship of one or more teeth when upper teeth are inside the lower teeth as a person bites down.

dark triangles—The dark, shadowy, triangular-shaped spaces between a person's teeth and at the widest corner of the lips when smiling fully. Also referred to as black buccal corridors, these indicate a narrow upper jaw.

DFO–dentofacial orthopedics—The use of oral treatment appliances for the purpose of reshaping facial structures to improve the health and appearance of an individual.

dyskinesia—Movement disorder that consists of the impairment of control over ordinary muscle movement and the presence of involuntary spasmodic movements or tics.

EMG–electromyography—A technique for evaluating and recording the electrical activity of muscle to determine its function and health.

epigenetic—Changes produced in biology caused by external mechanisms rather than genetic origins.

FFO–functional facial orthopedics—Similar to DFO, it is the use of oral treatment appliances for the purpose of reshaping, as well as repositioning, facial structures to improve the health and appearance of an individual.

fluorosis—A condition caused by excessive ingestion of fluorine resulting in mottling of the teeth and damage to the bones.

malocclusion—Literally means "bad bite" and exists when the upper and lower teeth are out of alignment with each other.

mandible—The lower jawbone containing the lower set of teeth.

mandibular—Pertaining to or the nature of the lower jawbone.

mandibular orthotic—An oral appliance worn on the lower teeth to reposition the lower jaw in order to correct a TMJ dysfunction.

maxilla—The upper jawbone structure that contains the upper teeth.

maxillary—Pertaining to the upper jawbone.

myocentric orthotic—An orthotic placed on the lower teeth and positioned so that when the teeth bite together the muscles are in their most balanced and ideal functional state.

myofunctional therapy—The specialty of medicine that evaluates and treats muscle disorders and habits that disrupt normal dental development.

myomonitor—A type of TENS that delivers a controlled, periodic electrical stimulation that is quite effective in relaxing muscles and reducing EMG readings to normal. It also increases blood circulation and range of motion allowing affected muscles to achieve normal resting length.

NPO–nasopharyngeal obstruction—Any obstacle within the nasal passageway that prevents the free flow of air when a person is breathing.

orofacial myology—The specialty of medicine that evaluates and treats a variety of oral and facial (orofacial) disorders and habits that disrupt normal dental development.

orthodontics—The branch of dentistry specializing in the prevention and correction of irregularities of the teeth.

OSA–obstructive sleep apnea—The most common type of sleep apnea, it is caused by obstruction of the airway behind the tongue when breathing while sleeping. It is characterized by repetitive pauses in breathing called apneas (literally, "without breath"), which by definition last at least ten seconds and result in loud, erratic snoring sounds. Also known as obstructive sleep apnea syndrome.

osteogenetic orthodontics—Orthodontics which incorporates accelerated methods for changing the bone structure to produce movements of the teeth.

otolaryngology—The specialty of medicine that deals with the anatomy, function, and diseases of the ear, nose, and throat.

overbite—An extension of the upper front teeth over the lower front teeth measured in millimeters when the mouth is closed. Also known as vertical overlap.

overjet—The horizontal projection of the upper front teeth beyond the lower front teeth when the mouth is closed. Also known as horizontal overlap.

polysomnogram–A sleep study done in a special laboratory to observe and measure sleep cycles and stages.

RLS–restless leg syndrome—A disorder in which there is an urge or need to move in an attempt to stop the creeping, unpleasant sensation in the legs and sometimes in the arms. This causes sleep disruption and daytime sleepiness.

RPE–rapid palatal expansion—This refers to a traditional orthodontic expansion appliance used to widen the upper jaw. It is attached to the teeth and usually activated daily by turning a screw to widen the upper jaw. The use of RPE is not advocated in this book.

SIDS–sudden infant death syndrome—A medical condition that causes a baby to die suddenly in his or her sleep.

SPE–slow palatal expansion—This refers to the slow activation (typically no faster than every third day) of a type of removable orthodontic appliance used to widen the upper jaw. This type of activation is advocated in this book.

stomatognathic system—The structures and all other connected anatomy in and around the mouth, jaw joints, and teeth that make up the chewing mechanism.

symmetry—The property of being the same or corresponding on both sides of a central dividing line. Harmony or beauty of form that results from balanced proportions.

TAD–temporary anchorage devices—Tiny implants screwed into an area of bone used as anchors to move teeth.

TENS–transcutanious electroneural stimulation—Low-voltage electrical impulses used to treat and relax muscles to achieve improved health. See also myomonitor.

TMD–temporomandibular dysfunction—Dysfunction within the TMJ (jaw joint) and associated structures within the head and neck.

TMJ–temporomandibular joint—The joint that facilitates movement of the lower jaw located between the condyle of the lower jaw and the temporal bone on each side of the head. Both joints act together when the jaw is moved.

traditional orthodontics—Orthodontic treatment methods as taught by most university graduate programs throughout the United States. These traditional methods include an emphasis on the use of braces (fixed appliances) to straighten teeth with little use of removable treatment appliances, which have been used predominately in Europe. A small number of university graduate programs in the United States do offer many of the treatment methods written about in this book.

underbite—Layman's slang for a malocclusion in which the lower teeth are outside the upper teeth when a person bites down.

Continuing Education and Speaking Engagements are Available

Educational opportunities for dentists to learn **The Lauson System: Nine Keys to Lower Facial Harmony** from Dr. Kent Lauson are available.

Dr. Lauson also is available to speak to general audiences regarding his treatment.

Those interested may contact the office at:

info@AuroraOrthodontics.com

or call us at 303.680.0020

www.AOTMJ.com
www.StraightTalkaboutCrookedTeeth.org

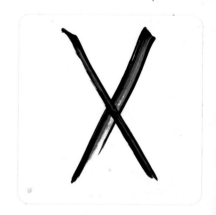